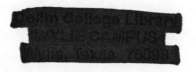

Restful
INSOMNIA

Restful INSOMNIA

HOW *to* GET *the* BENEFITS *of* SLEEP EVEN WHEN YOU CAN'T

Sondra Kornblatt

Author of *A Better Brain at Any Age*

Foreword by
Teresa E. Jacobs, MD

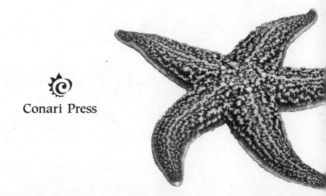

Conari Press

First published in 2010 by
Red Wheel/Weiser, LLC
With offices at:
500 Third Street, Suite 230
San Francisco, CA 94107
www.redwheelweiser.com

Library of Congress Cataloging-in-Publication Data
Kornblatt, Sondra.
Restful insomnia : how to get the benefits of sleep even when you can't /
Sondra Kornblatt.
p. cm.
ISBN 978-1-57324-467-1 (alk. paper)
1. Insomnia. 2. Sleep. 3. Rest. I. Title.
RC548.K67 2010
616.8'4982--dc22
2009031278

Cover design by Stewart Williams
Text design by Donna Linden
Typeset in English Grotesque, Miller Display, and Perpetua
Cover photographs: Waves on beach © MBPHOTO/iStockphoto.com;
Starfish © Dmitriy Kalinin/iStockphoto.com

Printed in Canada
TCP
10 9 8 7 6 5 4 3 2 1

The paper used in this publication meets the minimum requirements of
the American National Standard for Information Sciences—Permanence
of Paper for Printed Library Materials Z39.48-1992 (R1997).

Dedication

To Ragini Michaels: The only way I could explain *Restful Insomnia* was because of your teachings about paradox, identity, and being simultaneously spiritual and human. Thank you for helping me be (relatively) calm with your support on living life, not drama, connected to my Essence. May you be a happy and well rewarded Mystic in the Marketplace.

To three whom I wish could see this book:

My husband Howard: for your unwavering support of my writing *Restful Insomnia* (even though you didn't need it), and trust that it would help many lives. We all miss you.

Diane Rodriguez: for your steady and transforming presence. You were a fellow traveler of inner roads and outer reality. Thank you for accepting my quirks and supporting my strengths with a joyous heart.

Michael Pitrone: I have not begun to grieve you, my nearly lifelong friend. I'm still waiting for you to get back from Italy-in-the-sky, so I can tell you the latest, laugh at despair, sing Jennifer Warnes, and argue about the Right Use of Will. I dreamt last night about editing your head. . . . What does that mean? You grew up, but never grew old.

I love you all, and am so blessed to have you in my life.

Contents

Acknowledgments

MY ACKNOWLEDGEMENTS ARE A PARTY, and you, dear reader, are the guest of honor. Come on in, let me introduce you to these energizing and loving people who have supported my Restful Insomnia journey for almost ten years.

In the living room are my writing companions: Jodi Forschmeidt (who helped with editing and kept my writing down-to-earth), Michael Pitrone, author Ann Gonzales, Louisa's writing group, Ragini Michaels, Teresa Dahl, Irene Alexander, MJ Ryan, Jacque Boyd, writing teacher Priscilla Long, and my smart coworkers at Group Health. Thanks to my caring agent, who presented my proposal to those big New York publishers—and thanks to them for refusing, because those three years made me and the program much stronger. And thank you to Conari Press, from the editors Caroline Pincus and Jan Johnson, plus the bright publicity from Bonni Hamilton and Allyson May. I couldn't have asked for a better publisher.

To honor how much writing I did in their coffee shops, all these folks are drinking Starbucks coffee. I didn't learn how to get on their Internet, which kept my productivity high.

On the stairs you can see my clients and students from the past eight years. They've taught me the commonalities and individual quirks of insomnia, as well as how the techniques have worked during their nights. Their stories (with names changed) illustrate the points in the book.

In the hall are medically wise people chatting about health: avant-garde sleep doctors Teresa Jacobs, Ron Green, and Suzanne Krell who supported my Restful Insomnia program early on; Kathe Wallace, who reframed my view on getting up at night; Carrie Lafferty, who reframed my experience of my body; Fernando Vega and Sheldon Goldberg, doctors and humans extraordinaire.

Let's grab something to eat in the dining room, so I can introduce you to my friends. The PEPS families, who've been meeting for seventeen years since our eldest were born: I could not have gotten through this first (plus) year after Howard's death without you—not to mention the sixteen prior years. The Paradox Soiree: your wisdom, laughter, and togetherness make the journey of being alone more peaceful. Scott Caldwell, Evan Kentop, Greg Schroder, Billy and Sarah Pitrone: your presence carries new connections and brings back the essences of Diane, Howard, and Michael. And to those whose names have slipped at the moment (it's past my bedtime and this is past due), I appreciate you.

Finally, my families are crowded in the kitchen: To Nancy, Robert (I'll give this book to you on your 100th birthday in 2010), Lieschan and Piotr, Robert and Tanya, Jo, Colleen, Karen, and nieces and nephews, who make every get-together a celebration. To my parents, David and Barbara, whose pride and support allowed me to explore new grounds; to Rebecca and Henry for your caring by heart and by phone; to Anne for listening to my endless stories of woe, supporting my writing, and engaging in gmail chats on the difference between poo and poop; to nieces and nephews and legal or illegal partners who are most generally amusing. And deep affection for Milo and Ella, who took the bus, ate frozen pizza (cooked) with no veggies for many dinners, tolerated missing me at games and mealtimes, and still cheered each completed chapter. I love you.

Time to pop open some champagne and celebrate these amazing human lives and the birth of this book. Thank you, thank you all! Let's party!

Foreword

IT IS UNAVOIDABLE: every living creature needs sleep. Insomnia refers to the inability to get enough sleep to feel rested the next day. It can be described several ways: acute or chronic, trouble falling asleep or staying asleep, or waking too early. Some people have more than one form of insomnia, and overall it affects one third of adults at some point during a year. Insomnia can be a disorder in its own right, one which doctors and scientists know little about, but often it is a symptom of some other medical or psychological condition. In order for any treatment of insomnia to be effective, these other conditions must be evaluated and either ruled out or treated.

Insomnia can be an exasperating condition for both sufferers and those helping with treatment. Sleeping pills are often effective but are not the right choice for many, and most patients do not want to be on medicines for a long time. Habit changes (e.g., sleep hygiene, stimulus control, sleep restriction) can be very effective, but take patience, repetition, and, for many, are frustratingly difficult. Cognitive behavioral therapy for insomnia (CBTI) addresses some of the unpleasant thoughts about getting a good night's sleep that can aggravate insomnia.

In this book, *Restful Insomnia,* Sondra Kornblatt describes her journey not to cure but to manage her insomnia. She outlines the basic medical issues that can impact sleep and reviews the traditional approaches to treating insomnia. The central focus then emerges as she explores, often with step-by-step instructions, the details of her program of resting with insomnia. While many of her suggestions overlap with the traditional insomnia recommendations, she goes further to combine attention to the mind, the body, and the spirit to achieve rest. Her ability to clearly explain how to incorporate the techniques into one's sleep habits is what sets this book apart.

Ultimately, once medical conditions are excluded, a sleep specialist's goal is to help an insomnia sufferer function well during the day and not feel stressed about the sleep or lack of it at night. Sondra's program is a valuable addition to the approaches that I review with patients. Her book can help those with frequent insomnia explore different techniques at their own pace and focus on the ones that seem most beneficial. Everyone deserves a peaceful night; *Restful Insomnia* is one tool that will help many achieve it.

—Teresa E. Jacobs, MD
Creekside Sleep Medicine Center
Bellevue, Washington

Introduction: An Endarkened Insomniac Sees the Light

When I woke up this morning my girlfriend asked me,
"Did you sleep well?" I said, "No, I made a few mistakes."
—Steven Wright, comedian

I LOVE TO SLEEP.

I love to stretch out on smooth sheets, read by a dimmed lamp, and nestle into a soft pillow. Activity is left behind as I ride night dreams in a dark room and quiet house. I love waking to a new day—possibility, promise, and release from yesterday's irritations.

No surprise, then, that I hated insomnia—especially when chronic insomnia gripped me several years ago. I hated the rumpled sheets, flattened pillow, achy neck, and watching the clock in those hazy, dark hours between two and five. I hated rising in the morning with an empty tank—irritable and dreading the busy day, longing to close my eyes and rest.

Sure, I loved sleep, but did it love me? Some nights it did. But really, it was a fickle lover that promised bliss for eight hours—and then ran off.

I tried to seduce sleep. Pills had side effects: I was groggy, dependent, and duller during the day—and that didn't count the side effects of newer pills such as "sleep-driving" at night. Instead, I tried cures from books, Internet sites, acupuncturists, friends, and doctors. If they worked at all, it was just for a night or two. (However, various techniques work for some Restful Insomnia clients of mine. After developing the program, I began in 2003 to teach and coach clients in these techniques.) For me, all they did was give insomnia a slightly different twist:

- A snack or a glass of wine before bed (weight-gain insomnia)
- No food or wine after 8 P.M. (weight-loss insomnia)
- Sleepytime tea (wake-up-to-pee insomnia)
- Calcium, magnesium, melatonin, and L-tryptophan (expensive urine insomnia)
- Sleep "hygiene": lights-out at eleven, no napping, and waking at seven (exhausted insomnia)
- New pillow and mattress (in-debt insomnia)
- Exercise, warm baths, and relaxation exercises (healthy insomnia)
- Washing dishes, answering e-mail, and folding clothes (efficient and more exhausting insomnia)
- Yoga handstands, journal entries of irritations, banging my head against the headboard (*Help me!* insomnia)

It turns out the failed insomnia cures were gifts in disguise.

During those long, lonely nights, I uncovered riches in the dark—how to befriend myself at night, how to mimic the benefits of sleep, and how to create a deep rest that renewed me. I shared these methods with other insomniacs who learned to uncover their own riches and rest in the dark.

In this book, I'm excited to share my Restful Insomnia program with you, one of the seventy million Americans who battle insomnia each night. This book covers how you can:

- Create restful waking hours
- Calm the restless mind
- Connect with your body to release stress
- Mimic the benefits of sleep—and greet the morning refreshed

You'll learn the five steps of the Restful Insomnia program along with specific ways to create a comforting space, get in tune with dusk at night, let go of relentless thoughts, reduce the charge of emotions, and connect to a larger perspective on problems and the joy of life.

Let's start with how I went from hating insomnia to . . . OK, not loving it, but valuing it, and accepting the gifts that can help everyone's nights.

Grieving and Accepting Insomnia

Before I began accepting the gifts, I suffered.

During my bout of chronic insomnia, I was cranky and fuzzy in the morning, a sour space cadet during the

day, and depressed in the evening because that fickle lover Sleep would probably not show. Nights were spirals of tension when I longed for sleep. Insomniac life was like driving with a piston missing—chugging and groaning through days and nights.

I longed for sleep so much, I grieved not having it. In fact, I went through the typical five stages of grief.

Denial: "Lots of people do OK on a couple hours of sleep. I'm *fine!*"

Anger: "Why is that light red? Who moved my Kleenex box? Nobody cares about me."

Bargaining: "Maybe if I mop the kitchen floor, I'll be able to sleep."

Depression: "I'll never sleep. I'll never be able to work, think, or get anything done. Life is hopeless."

Acceptance: "OK, here's insomnia. How can I learn to make the best of it?"

Acceptance came (and still comes) in small "aha" moments. It allowed me to look at sleeplessness in a new way, to uncover what *really* happened at night.

Acceptance

Acceptance of insomnia first came during the day.

I was walking with a friend and whining about being tired, not being able to sleep, and needing a couple of

hours to myself—away from the kids, work, and errands. As I grumbled, a voice in my head whispered, "Three A.M." I realized I could have my hours to myself—when I couldn't sleep. While I wanted that time during the day, twelve hours earlier (What else was I doing in those early hours?), I was too exhausted to be productive, and moaning didn't make me happy—nor make me feel rested. So the next few nights at 3 A.M., I pretended I was having a few dark hours alone during the day: I visualized my success, wrote in my journal, and practiced talking gently to myself.

That was the beginning of exploring insomnia in a new way—with acceptance.

Instead of *thinking* about insomnia (and fixing it), I felt it. Which meant I experienced my body and how the mind, emotions, body habits, environment, and the night itself affected my ability to sleep. I realized that my Conscious Mind (my thinking, planning, fixing mind) kept me awake at night, and that my Unconscious Mind (responsible for body connection, intuition, dreaminess) led me to rest.

When I stopped fighting insomnia and focused on my Unconscious Mind, I developed ways to soothe my body, mind, emotions, and environment. And those techniques, or variations on them, worked night after night.

Some nights, I rested deeply. Some nights, I fell asleep. Either way, I was happy to find that insomnia was no longer a big problem. I discovered that I was mimicking the benefits of sleep and greeting the mornings refreshed, with more productive days.

The Five Steps of Restful Insomnia

I talked with others about Restful Insomnia and came across many insomniacs tired of hating sleepless nights. I started teaching them my techniques in classes and one-on-one, and my clients loved it. Some changed their insomnia just by looking at sleeplessness in a new way. (*Hey, I can relax if I don't have to make myself sleep!*) However, most of us need a plan when we're lost in insomniac tension. After all, we've spent many nights—even decades—in the sleepless struggle.

Five steps organize the Restful Insomnia techniques that help you enjoy your nights:

1. Create a soothing night environment
2. Befriend the body
3. Diminish the thinking mind
4. Release the hold of emotions
5. Tap into the natural or spiritual self

Each step includes specific methods you can use tonight to change your body, mind, emotions, and spirit when you can't sleep. Each chapter relates to the five steps, after introducing the basic Restful Insomnia concepts, in this way:

1. Create a soothing night environment (*Creating a Night Nest; Evening Rituals*)
2. Befriend the body (*Getting into Your Body; Night Yoga; A New Relationship with Pain and Discomfort*)

3. Diminish the thinking mind (*Change Your Mind; Resting with Meditation*)
4. Release the hold of emotions (*Emotions and Touch; Wisdom Writing*)
5. Tap into the natural or spiritual self (*Finding Your Spiritual Center; Grounding; Positive Focus*)

The book ends with a chapter on *Taking Restful Insomnia Insights into Sleep and the Day.*

Here's a summary of how the steps work:

To *create a soothing night environment,* you can use Evening Rituals to welcome the dark, and gather a Night Nest stash; to *befriend the body,* you can focus on the wisdom of body sensations or release tension with Night Yoga; you can *diminish the thinking mind* by understanding how the Conscious Mind keeps you awake and how the Unconscious Mind helps you rest; you can *release the hold of emotions* by using acupressure tapping techniques and Wisdom Writing; and you can *tap into the natural or spiritual self* through visualization, being aware of body sensation, and meditation.

The five-step path brings you back to a calm state at night.

Once you're aware of the ways to relax, you can choose the best Restful Insomnia techniques for you. These techniques may change from night to night and season to season.

Although I no longer have the same chronic insomnia of four to five nights a week, I still have plenty of sleepless hours—in the middle of the night or when I try to fall asleep. Even now, when sleeplessness sneaks back after a few good nights of sleep, I might have moments of insomnia resentment. (*You again? I didn't miss you.*) Then I remember Restful Insomnia and practice my current favorite techniques. Right now they include rolling my eyes down (see chapter 6, "Getting into Your Body") and pausing at the edge of each inhale and exhale (see chapter 10, "Resting with Meditation"). Or I go back to the foundation of the five-step program: darken the environment, notice the body, tap acupressure points to soothe emotions, discharge problems with Wisdom Writing, and connect to the spiritual self.

I've gotten many gifts from insomnia: The first was learning how to accept sleeplessness as part of life and using it to rest and find renewal. Then I found gifts within Restful Insomnia, from insights about myself to healing visualizations and listening to my husband talk in his sleep. None of these gifts would I return, even if I had a receipt.

Sleep and Renewal

I still love to sleep, letting my mind just turn off.

But now I like insomnia, too. I experience my body, learn that my emotions aren't the whole truth, and touch into deeper wisdom. I connect with the essence of night's rejuvenation.

During the day, I take the perspectives I uncover during Restful Insomnia to keep me focused, relaxed, creative, and connected to a larger perspective on life, even as I hurry on errands or make dinner.

The journey of insomnia led me to new roads I wouldn't change. Let me show you how you can befriend the night—and your life.

Chapter 1

The Conscious Mind and the Unconscious Mind— Who's Driving the Van?

It is the mind that makes the body.
—Sojourner Truth

MY CLIENT TOM BRUSHED HIS TEETH, put on his red plaid flannel PJs, and snuggled under the comforter next to his sleeping wife. He was definitely ready for bed after a long day at his insurance business. He tried to read *Master and Commander*, which he loved when he was younger, but he was too sleepy to get through the first chapter. *It'll be a good weekend read,* he thought as he turned off the lamp.

Tom's eyes closed as he listened to Linda's breathing. Quiet, dark, restful . . . *Terrific, I'm falling asleep.* His thoughts drifted to gardening, his next surfing adventure, his upcoming anniversary as he settled into the bed.

Shoot! He forgot to call the landlord to renegotiate the lease. The payment for quarterly taxes was due tomorrow. They had a teacher conference for their daughter at three fifteen, right before his team meeting at four.

Needless to say, Tom's eyes were no longer closed. He was too tired to turn the lamp back on, and there was really nothing to do tonight about anything. So he lay in bed and wondered whether the negotiation strategies on his desk covered all the bases, if they should talk to the teacher about that girl bullying their daughter, and if he needed to transfer money from his savings for the taxes.

His body wanted to sleep, but his mind had taken over. Actually, it was his Conscious Mind that took over, focused on getting things done, just like it did during the day.

Letting Go of the Restless Mind

You probably know that your mind can keep you from rest at night—especially if you've been kept awake by the "restless mind" touted in pharmaceutical ads. However, with Restful Insomnia you have more options than medicine to let you and your mind rest.

This book is about those options, about how to step aside from the Conscious Mind at night and focus instead on the restful dreaminess of the Unconscious Mind. Unfortunately, there is no on-off mind switch (other than sleep or anesthesia). However, you can invite this shift of focus; it just takes practice.

This chapter clarifies my definition of the Conscious Mind and the Unconscious Mind. It also talks about how the Conscious Mind takes charge during the day while the Unconscious Mind takes over at night—and how that affects the body.

The Conscious Mind and the Unconscious Mind

You listen to your chattering mind all day and many restless nights. It chatters off orders, concerns, plans, and analyses even if your body's pooped: "You didn't finish the bills today; You should decide this quarter's strategy after you read the marketing report; Go to sleep already!"

That chattering mind is your Conscious Mind. It thrives on being productive and in charge. It has goals, connects us with our community, and follows and creates rules.

The Conscious Mind is convinced that it's the boss, the head honcho, the one-and-only chief. This is especially true during insomnia, when it ignores the other side: the wisdom of the Unconscious Mind.

The Unconscious Mind is a storehouse that holds your experiences, memories, beliefs, and desires. It communicates in images, sounds, dialogues, smells, textures, and sensations. The Unconscious Mind generates dreams, creativity, and intuition as well as automatic body processes, such as blinking and breathing. It shapes your perception of reality and underlies your beliefs about life and yourself.

Imagine life with just the Conscious Mind: we're robots without creativity or a heart. Imagine life with just the Unconscious Mind: we're lost, like Alzheimer's patients. There's a natural balance between the Conscious Mind and the Unconscious Mind, and between the cycles of day and night.

During the day, the Conscious Mind holds court. I see the Conscious Mind driving a minivan—full of kids, a briefcase, dry cleaning, groceries, sports equipment, and a to-do list trailing out the window.

The Conscious Mind doesn't drive alone, though. Sitting in the passenger seat is the Unconscious Mind—navigating. It suggests paths to follow, connects the tasks to a bigger picture, and may create obstacles (if the plan doesn't meet familiar beliefs). The Unconscious Mind is actually guiding the van—but let's keep that a secret from the Conscious Mind.

At night, the balance changes: the Conscious Mind rests, and the Unconscious Mind leads. The Unconscious Mind leaves the minivan behind to guide a sturdy raft through moonlit water. It tells stories of the day to the sleepy Conscious Mind—odd stories filled with experiences from the day and from years before, images from movies and emotions, and perhaps possibilities for the future.

Restful Insomnia

The raft floats to islands where it drops off old baggage and gathers new information. The night journey cleans the slate and then prepares the Conscious Mind for tomorrow.

In sleep we transform from the minivan to the raft, from to-do tension to dreamy relaxation. But in insomnia, we don't let go. The Conscious Mind—the restless mind—demands order and organization, just as it does during the day.

Restful Insomnia techniques help your Conscious Mind rest so you can follow the dreamy and creative Unconscious Mind. You're mimicking the natural pathway from day to night, allowing the mind and body to balance and renew.

Balance of the Minds

Here's how I discovered the mind-body balance during my many sleepless hours

I explored the body's perspective on insomnia. I started with the different body sensations that resulted from physical stimuli (caffeine, hormones, or too long a nap during the day). Next I explored where I experienced emotional states (anger in the jaw, fear in the stomach, sadness in the chest). Then I explored how different mental states changed my body as well.

Here's an example. My husband and I were quarrelling, except he was asleep and I had the full-blown quarrel in my head. I kept going over the argument again and again, on a quest to find the perfect zinger. One where he'd say, "You're right, I'm sorry. I'll change." Unfortunately, the husband in my head kept defeating my zingers with new responses, and there I was: awake in the mental pinball machine of impossible resolution. (You can learn more about situations like this one in chapter 9, "Change Your Mind.")

Then I heard acceptance whisper, "Your mind is stuck. Focus on your body."

Hell, no. I wanted to fix my husband, not me. Still, I hated being awake. *All right, I'll try.* To change direction was like steering a semitruck after the front tires blew out.

My body . . . I know I have one. Inhale. I noticed how my stomach clenched, my teeth locked, my hands curled. *Exhale.* The tension around my heart loosened a millimeter . . . a little space around the rage. My body sensations kept shifting and moving. I felt like I was watching an anger aquarium in my body. Look, a spitting-mad tetra . . . the not-my-fault carp . . . the you-forget-stuff-too hatchet fish.

I rested into dreamy odd sensations and let my body experience the anger without trying to fix it. *I think I'm falling asleep.*

My mental alarm clock went off. *Now I'm not falling asleep. I was so close. . . . I should just get up and answer my old e-mail or pay the bills.*

What was the reaction to my buzzing mind? I felt my head, like it was buzzing, like the sensation you get after you rub your palms briskly together. My brain was charged like a halogen bulb on high.

Weird and curious. Did thinking I'm falling asleep make my head buzz and wake me up? In that moment, I realized that insomnia was being driven by my thoughts, and Restful Insomnia started by my thoughts and paying attention to my body.

I had a lot of time to explore how the Conscious Mind and the Unconscious Mind work. Like how the Conscious Mind can chase the connection to sleep away. Or how to step aside from the Conscious Mind. I discovered that altering the relationship with one's mind is a key to soothing the body at night. I could see it in my husband.

The Minds of Restful Insomnia

My husband was great at letting go of the Conscious Mind at night. If something bugged him, he'd just figure that the problem would get resolved in some way, somehow, someday—and fall asleep.

However, for me, and for many of my clients, the Conscious Mind is too active at night to just stop thinking, worrying, and planning. It needs something to replace its manic anxiety and help it fall back behind the Unconscious Mind. The Restful Insomnia techniques use the environment, the body, emotions, spiritual views, and new mental perspectives to change the mind in the middle of the night.

Here are some examples of these techniques, described fully later in the book:

- Distract the Conscious Mind by counting sheep—or blessings.
- Do a relaxation exercise, but *not* to fall asleep. Instead, relax to appreciate the body at night.
- Create a soothing stash of items with a Night Nest. (See chapter 4, "Creating a Night Nest.")
- Develop a body-focused Evening Ritual—a habit to help your body remember the dusk. (See chapter 5, "Evening Rituals.")

The Conscious Mind may resist at first—remember, its job is to be in charge and plan, worry, and think. Over time, though, it will find that the Unconscious Mind really helps it solve problems, change, and accept the unexpected.

Your Conscious Mind Learns

When my client Tom started looking for techniques to help him bring his Unconscious Mind to the fore, his Conscious Mind said, "Hell no, I'm in charge, and I can do what needs to be done." However, Tom's Conscious Mind started to sense that the Unconscious Mind actually *helped* it function better, and his body started to rest.

In the following chapters, I will show you techniques that re-adjust the balance between your Conscious Mind

and your Unconscious Mind so that you can rest and renew during the night.

Chapter 2

What's the Problem?

Insomnia: a contagious disease often
transmitted from babies to parents.
—Shannon Fife

MY FRIEND MALLORY went to an acupuncturist one day for help with a long bout of insomnia. The acupuncturist, Dr. Chen, held her fingers on Mallory's pulses for over a minute and then inspected her tongue, top and bottom. Dr. Chen looked for causes of insomnia—weak liver, heart, or spleen meridians—not recognized in the traditional Western perspective. Homeopaths also look for subtle symptoms of insomnia such as time of insomnia, chills, stress, visions, and more. Whatever approach, something is keeping your natural ability to sleep or rest off your radar. Identifying the causes, even if there's nothing to be done about them, helps you understand who you are in the night. Who you are, combined with your environment, food intake, ability to breathe, tension, allergies, medicine, and other things that may interrupt your sleep.

It's helpful to know you have considerable sleepless company. Prescriptions for sleeping pills have increased by 60 percent in six years. Luxury mattresses sell for ten to twenty thousand dollars. One-third of American adults have trouble falling or staying asleep, and of those, half, or more than thirty-five million, have chronic insomnia, defined as poor sleep every night or most nights, according to the National Sleep Foundation. More women than men have insomnia, and its incidence increases as the population ages. Insomnia affects exhausted drivers, salesclerks, and coworkers.

This chapter describes the medical view of insomnia, together with suggested traditional and alternative cures. (If you *can* fix your insomnia, you might as well.) The chapter also explains how Restful Insomnia goes beyond medical remedies to help you change your relationship to sleepless nights. And it offers Restful Insomnia perspectives on some ignored causes of insomnia, from hunger to the gotta-do mind.

Once you have a better sense of what's going on at night, your mind can stop trying to figure it all out and get some rest.

What Is Insomnia?

"What is insomnia?" is a silly question for anyone who can't sleep. As French writer Marie de Rabutin-Chantal said, "There are twelve hours in the day, and more than fifty in the night."

However, it's helpful to understand how medicine, especially sleep medicine, defines the problem. (Sleep-medicine physicians, usually pulmonologists, focus on sleep issues ranging from breathing disorders to narcolepsy—falling asleep rapidly in daytime situations, such as driving.)

Sleep doctors describe three types of insomnia:

- **Transient insomnia** lasts only a night or two. It is usually caused by some outside influence—sleeping in a strange bed, perhaps in a hotel room; worrying about a big presentation you have to make in the morning; having trouble getting to sleep on Christmas Eve as a child.
- **Short-term insomnia** can last from a few days to a few weeks. Stress, poor sleep habits, premenstrual syndrome, or jet lag can bring this on. So can worry about things like health, business, and relationships.
- **Chronic insomnia** occurs many nights of the week. It may last for months or years and sometimes starts in early childhood. The resultant loss of sleep causes many health and cognitive problems.

As you know from your own experience, not getting enough sleep or rest creates problems like worsening moods and irritability; excessive daytime sleepiness; diminished coordination, memory, concentration, and decision-making ability; increased frequency of colds; and weight gain.

Although acupuncture and homeopathy identify alternative causes of insomnia, the traditional medical causes are these:

- **Physical ailments:** Breathing or muscle disorders such as sleep apnea or restless legs (unavoidable urge to shake or move legs or other body parts; more pronounced near bedtime), reflux, arthritis, asthma, allergies, and diabetes.
- **Environmental factors:** Interruptions, discomforts, jet lag, penetrating light, and sleep hygiene. (*Sleep hygiene* is a term created during the turn of the last century and means keeping regular sleeping hours.)
- **Emotional factors:** Stress, intense emotional reactions, depression, and psychiatric disorders.
- **Other factors:** Misuse of sleeping pills, use of stimulants, and side effects of medication.

Not sleeping may mean more than irritable nights and sleepy days. It could be a symptom of a larger health issue, and these are times that you should talk to your doctor.

- **Depression.** Insomnia is one of the most common symptoms of depression at any age. Some people hit a depressed wall a few months after a difficult situation or loss and don't realize they're still carrying the effects. Counseling and medication can ease the blues.

- **Thyroid problems.** Usually too much thyroid, but sleep cycles can be interrupted with too little thyroid as well.
- **Hypertension.** High blood pressure can be caused by and lead to a feeling of tension, contributing to insomnia.
- **Kidney disease, arthritis, , asthma, heart failure.** These conditions and treatments may make it hard to fall and stay asleep.
- **Sleep-wake-cycle disorder.** Your internal circadian rhythm is off.
- **Sleep apnea.** If you snore, if you've been told that you stop breathing for short periods during your sleep, or if you wake up tired even though you sleep through the night, you may have sleep apnea, which can be life threatening.
- **Other problems.** See your doctor if you experience excessive sleepiness during the day; if you find that you fall asleep at inappropriate moments (like when you're operating machinery such as electric saws, carving knives, or automobiles); if you have pain or uncomfortable "creepy" feelings in your legs (restless leg syndrome); or if you walk or make aggressive movements in your sleep. All of these may be related to medical conditions that can be treated by your physician.

What's the Problem?

Use your doctor to rule out—and treat—physical factors or medication interactions that may be making it harder for you to sleep. If your physician has not been trained in treating sleep disorders, ask for a referral.

The Promise of Insomnia Cures

How can you cure insomnia? Aerobic exercise before 8 P.M. might solve all your sleep problems. Or you may try all the remedies you've found in books and on the Internet, and still look up more on the Net in the middle of the night. Having recommended and experienced rounds of insomnia remedies, I've found they have individual success, just like individual orders at a coffee shop: you like a *grande* latte with caramel syrup on the bottom not stirred and nonfat dry-foam milk, and your friend likes herbal tea with no sugar. Same thing if you try an insomnia remedy such as calcium, sleep hygiene, or the Sleep Number bed. It might work for your best friend but not for you.

However, one of the following ideas might work for you. I've gathered them from my own exploration and from *www.Well.com*. While some of these contradict the Restful Insomnia perspective, there's more than one way to skin a cat. (*Yuck.* More than one way to *pet* a cat.)

- Take a warm bath.
- Get a massage. (I heard that Marilyn Monroe had a masseuse come every night before bedtime—I wish!)

- Listen to music.
- Drink warm milk.
- Drink herbal tea.
- Eat a bedtime snack.
- Stop eating after 8 P.M.
- Avoid caffeine, alcohol, and tobacco. (Caffeine can actually wake you up in the *middle* of the night, after you've had all the rest your jived-up body needs.)
- Sleep in a well-ventilated room.
- Sleep on a good, firm bed (or a not-so-firm bed, depending on your source).
- Sleep on your back. (That can make you snore, which might not bother you but will give your sleep partner insomnia.)
- Get some physical exercise during the day.
- Keep regular bedtime hours.
- If you can't sleep, get up (not part of the Restful Insomnia program).
- Don't sleep in.
- Get up earlier in the morning.
- Keep your bed a place only for sleep (to associate your bed with sleep, per behavior modification).
- Avoid naps.
- Avoid illuminated bedroom clocks (especially those with a green light).
- Sleep with your head facing north.
- Don't watch TV or hang out on the computer before going to bed. (A Japanese study found that computer games significantly increased insomnia.)

- Don't read before going to bed (advice not to be found in the Restful Insomnia book).
- Rub your stomach gently.
- Do a progressive relaxation exercise up or down your body.
- Breathe deeply.
- Have sexual pleasure.
- Visualize something peaceful.
- Visualize something boring.
- Imagine it's time to get up.
- Take L-tryptophan (it's in turkey), calcium, and/or magnesium.
- Stare at the ceiling until your eyes must close.

I hope you can find a way to sleep all night. But if not, the night is not lost.

Is Restful Insomnia an Alternative Cure?

Where does Restful Insomnia fit in with all these cures? It doesn't.

The Restful Insomnia approach is avant-garde, on the evolutionary edge of how to look at insomnia. To use a cliché, it involves a paradigm shift: Restful Insomnia doesn't see insomnia as a problem to get rid of. Instead, it sees it as a gift to make use of, and from which you get some of the benefits of sleep.

Some of the tips to help make Restful Insomnia work for you are the same as the remedies described earlier, such as breathing deeply (isn't that a cure for everything?); avoiding illuminated clocks, or at least turning them away from the bed; and sleeping in a well-ventilated room.

Some tips are unique to Restful Insomnia. Reading helps you follow your Unconscious Mind (assuming the material isn't upsetting) by providing images, sensations, and stories that come from the author's Unconscious Mind. Darkness and Evening Rituals help the body align with the cycle of activity and rest. So does *not worrying about falling asleep*—a contradiction to insomnia cures. Insomnia cures are based on the idea that insomnia is out-and-out bad and that a person *should* fall asleep no matter what. And simply worrying about falling asleep engages your Conscious Mind to direct an unconscious process.

Here are some Restful Insomnia perspectives and hints that help you minimize night stresses and maximize your ability to rest.

Peeing

My daughter laughs when I tell her to be careful of drinking tea too late at night in case she has to wake up to pee. "I don't have to pee in the middle of the night," she responds. "Only old people like you do." Unfortunately, she's right.

Physical therapist Kathe Wallace specializes in pelvic floor issues that affect urination, and her approach goes well beyond Kegel exercises (pulling the vaginal muscles in and up). She says our bladders are bigger than we think they are, but we've trained them to "pee just in case" for decades. One way to reduce the number of nighttime bathroom visits is to reduce the acidity in your food (from tomatoes, citrus, vinegar, coffee, tea, milk, cola, artificial sweeteners, etc.). Does drinking fewer liquids help? Actually, reduced fluids can make your urine more concentrated (dark yellow), which can irritate your bladder so you urinate more. It also encourages the growth of bacteria, which may lead to infections.

If you have a bladder infection, you need to pee often—very often, believe me. You may also have some irritation or a sensation of not finishing even after you're done. If you have these symptoms, see your doctor.

Other tips that may help lessen peeing at night:

• Cut back on evening alcohol
• No tea or coffee after 8 p.m. (or earlier)
• Reduce sugar and increase cranberry supplements

And finally, keep the path of your nightly trip to the bathroom as dark as you safely can, to keep your melatonin production going and your Conscious Mind from getting stimulated. Try using red bulbs in your night-lights.

Hormones

Estrogen swings—from premenstrual syndrome to menopause—and certain medications make women's sleep cycles irregular. There is a lot of advice about menopause and PMS, including changing diets, exercising, and taking supplements. Check out a few ideas to see how they work.

To soothe your nights with Restful Insomnia, start with stocking your Night Nest (see chapter 4) with comforting items. Could be a washcloth and an extra nightgown if you have a hot flash, Calms Forté (a homeopathic remedy that is calming), and water. And to deal with emotional intensity, try Energy Psychology and Wisdom Writing (see chapters 11 and 12, respectively).

Interruptions

"There is no snooze button on a cat who wants breakfast." Cats, babies, children, fire trucks, car alarms, wrong numbers, snoring spouses (the joke is, that's why most menopausal women can't sleep), late teenage curfew— all reasons we get roused from our slumber. But interruptions cause fewer problems with Restful Insomnia:

1. **Timing.** Most people sleep in ninety-minute cycles. Interruptions at certain times (for me, it's within the first twenty minutes) can disrupt the body's flow toward sleep. What to do? Stay horizontal, disengage the Conscious Mind, and use Restful Insomnia tips to remind your body that it can "pick up the lost stitch" and return to deep rest or sleep.

2. **Irritation.** Any of the techniques in chapter 11, "Emotions and Touch," or in the blame section in chapter 9, "Change your Mind," will help give a little

distance from the annoyance of being *needlessly* interrupted. You can also connect with your Spiritual Center, to accept what is.

3. **Sensitivity.** The white-noise machine reduces the intensity of interruptions by reducing the contrast of
sounds. If you imagine sound as an image, high contrast is
a black-and-white picture (a ringing phone sounds loud
in the silence); lower contrast is a black picture on a gray
background (a ringing phone doesn't sound as loud with
white noise). Fans and other white noise devices are a
healthy alternative to sleeping pills, says Dr. Beth Malow,
professor of neurology at Vanderbilt University.

Gotta-do Mind

As you rest at night, all the gotta-dos that were on the
back burner during the day can explode in your head.
Work to-dos (meetings, agendas, résumés), house to-dos
(broken burner on the stove, oak leaves in the yard), family to-dos (baseball snacks, orthodontist appointments)—
they all make the Conscious Mind so excited. For some,
writing these down on a list (in a dim location) will let the
Conscious Mind release. For others, each item added to
the list makes you want to get up and get something done.
You'll be more productive tomorrow if you have a night
of rest first:

*   Create a structure so your Conscious Mind can let
    go: write a list, use mnemonics to remember the key
    points, or jot a bullet-point outline of your job skills.

- Focus on your body. Let your attention float—and return to —your skin, stomach, breathing, throat. Imagine colors, sounds, or sensations if that calms you.
- Ask yourself (consult your body wisdom) why you're feeling the urgency now. Perhaps part of you identifies with being "good," or with fixing a problem. Use some Energy Psychology, your Spiritual Center, or Wisdom Writing to envision possibilities of a relaxed life.

Hunger

I had a client who went to bed at 2, 3, or 4 A.M. and woke at eleven or noon. It's a good thing she was retired, because even when she was working and had to be at work at ten, she had trouble making it on time. How did her hunger affect her sleep? She'd get hungry at bedtime, so she'd delay going to bed so she could have a snack, thus waking up later in the mornings.

Hunger is an important signal for food during the day. At night, though, your liver will provide the glucose your body needs to make it through the night, according to University of Washington nutritionist Dori Khakpour. That's why you're not usually starving when you wake in the morning. So relax—the hunger pangs usually go away and your body knows how to make it through the night.

Creativity Storms

When you're resting and dreamy, your brain comes up with new and wonderful ideas—the design for a sweater, a historical novel complete with all the characters, the perfect organizer to fix the mess in the closet. What a gift. You can't help but want to run to a computer, paper, or easel to catch it.

Not a great partner of sleep or rest.

I'm not suggesting you throw the baby out with the bathwater and ignore your nighttime ideas. I'm suggesting that you widen your options:

- Sit and write with a dim light or lighted pen. Write the whole thing, if that feels right, or use bullet points or make sketches to remind you of your ideas when you're more awake.
- Use mnemonics to remember key points, which I did when I wanted to remember to add the word *hunger* to this chapter. I saw the chapter title with a big blue letter *H* hanging from the *W* in "What's the Problem?" In the morning, I remembered the letter, and the concept came a few minutes later.
- Check out whether you're identifying with the creative streak, as in "I'm special, I'll be famous, I'll be on *Oprah.*" That takes you away from the essence of creativity, because you're in the future, not the present.
- Acknowledge that you're the receptacle of the inspiration, not the source. Then you recognize, as a friend says, that "a brushstroke of the divine came through me."
- Appreciate the gift, and, just like when someone hands you a wrapped present, you can decide if now is the time to accept it. When someone hands you a present as you're

draining hot pasta in the sink, you might say, "Thank you. I can't accept it right now, but I'd like it later."

Why Are You Up?

Acupuncture helped Mallory with her insomnia, but not all the time. She came to me because she wanted to identify possible root causes for her sleeplessness. I helped her dig beneath the label of "can't sleep" and had her answer these questions, which can also help you:

1. What are your usual nightly and sleeping habits—bedtimes, waking times, activities before sleep, and so forth?
2. What's your sleeping environment like?
3. When did your insomnia start? How many nights per week does it affect you?
4. Did anything significant happen at that time, in your environment—medication, health, or stress?
5. Are there times when insomnia is worse or better than others?
6. What do you do when you can't sleep?
7. If you have a restless mind, what do you think about at night?
8. Are there particular emotions that arise during insomnia?
9. What do you do during insomnia? Do you watch TV or use the computer?

10. What's the worst part of your insomnia?
11. What do you do that helps?

What to Do Tonight

When you're sleepless, notice where your energy goes—tension in your stomach, buzzing in your head, clenching in your jaw. Your body wisdom can give you clues as to whether you're awake due to stress, physical health, even caffeine. Notice and learn from where the sensations move in your body. You may be on your way to changing how you relate to sleep before you even close your eyes.

Chapter 3

Reframing and Using Insomnia

*The real voyage of discovery consists not in
seeking new landscapes, but in having new eyes.*
—Marcel Proust

INSOMNIA WINS OR YOU WIN.

That's how most insomniacs view the nights: a lonely
battle with sleeplessness, the diabolical enemy. You can
gather combat forces, but it's hard to outwit insomnia. You
need a modern John Wayne who strides into your bedroom and proclaims: "Insomnia, this bed ain't big enough
for both of us, so get outta here by sundown."

OK, so that only works in the movies.

But there is a hero in real life—you. You can rescue yourself, if not from the sleep poacher, at least from

suffering with it. It starts with reframing—changing how you view insomnia.

Reframing means looking at something from a new perspective. You do it all the time. When you look at the famous optical illusion and see a vase, then two profiles, you've changed how you're seeing the picture. When you flinch at a bug and then find that it's a piece of lint, you've changed how you're looking at your environment. When you groan over your dog's failed house-training only to learn that your roommate spilled lemonade, you're putting a new frame around what's actually there, and it becomes a different experience.

Students realize they've framed their lives when I mention reframing in class. Rachel, for instance, remembered a disappointing reframing that occurred while beach-combing on the Oregon coast. She had climbed down the grassy dunes to the gray sandy beach, ribbons of white breakers and her kids in the distance. Rachel looked for treasures peeping out under tire tracks and footprints in the sand. She hoped to spy a whole sand dollar or a pretty shell to show the kids. Mostly she found seagull feathers, red burned sparklers, crab backs, crab claws, and a million broken sand dollars.

Then the sun glinted off a smooth, white, opaque shape under some kelp. Maybe it was quartz or a moonstone. She leaned over to pick it up, drawn by its cool, dense shape.

Once her fingers touched it, she knew that it wasn't a pebble—it was slick, light, and a perfect cylinder: a film canister. The treasure became trash.

The object never changed, but Rachel's expectations did. The smooth, white, round object turned from beautiful to ugly just by what she thought. In the Restful Insomnia class, Rachel realized that if her mind could create disappointment, it might also reframe things so that she could see opportunities and support.

Framing and Reframing

Creating frames of reference is a natural function of the mind, sorting perceptions into categories to make sense of the environment. It's shorthand for processing information so you don't have to analyze each item every time you see it. Framing allows you to quickly decide that a peripheral moving blur might be a bicyclist and slam on the brakes.

Toddlers create frames of reference as they develop and refine categories. My son identified animals, then reptiles; balls, then apples; things that move, then trucks. Soon he created his own categories: cars with curved backs (VW beetles, older Saabs, a 1948 Dodge) became "turtle cars." His language reflected how he framed things.

Your language reflects the categories you construct for objects, events, and interactions. However, frames remain invisible unless you pay attention to them. Like eyeglasses, you see through them but forget they're framing your vision.

Reframing—becoming aware of your eyeglasses—is also a natural function. You notice your perspective, try on new viewpoints, and change your relationship to a situation. And in doing so, you change how you relate to your life.

How to Reframe

If life gives you lemons, make lemonade. That's the reframing cliché. Some people think that means living a Pollyanna life or becoming a born-again optimist. Instead, reframing adds a larger horizon to focus on, even when sadness or uncomfortable feelings remain.

Here's how to find the sugar to sweeten up sour lemons:

Multiple perspectives: See your problem from different viewpoints; try moving to new angles—physically, if possible.

To reframe during the day (which can help your nights), stand up and describe or write what you struggle with—for example, you're irritated with your girlfriend's spoiled cat. Take a step to move to a new location and describe your as-usual relationship to the problem. Could be that you're jealous that she treats the cat better than you. Next, move to a different point, as if you're going in a circle around the problem, and describe a new way to react; continue doing this at different points in the circle.

In one description, you might cuddle up to the cat. (I know, you're not a cat person—but you can pretend, to gain the new view.) In another, you imagine you're a dog. Move into a corner (cat phobia) or up on a chair looking down. If you can't think of different perspectives, pretend you are someone or something else—the Dalai Lama, PETA, or the stars. You might find a way to accept your girlfriend's furball.

To reframe during Restful Insomnia, try some small physical movements if you can. Turn your head, move your body, or position your hands to represent new perspectives; draw images of perspectives on a paper; or use finger puppets. (See chapter 6, "Getting into Your Body.")

After you've experienced these new perspectives, focus on the one that gives you the most leeway and options—a positive reframe.

Humor: How many comics hang on your fridge? They're a positive reframe of something that's irritating— the more irritating, the funnier the comic. On my fridge is a comic from "Candorville," showing Susan awake in bed at two in the morning. She's reading *The Joy of Sleep.*

Humor has many benefits, including replacing the familiar with the unexpected so you can laugh at things that bother you. That's why dark humor has a strong pull, if it has the right timing.

To reframe something that bothers you with humor, find something in your situation that's amusing. With the conceited cat, laugh at how the cat is more of a princess than your girlfriend. If you're sick of office life, check out the Cube dolls from Archie McPhees. If your computer still doesn't paste what you've copied—again!—rename it a monitor potato or paste an ugly face on it when you leave for the day.

If you've lose your sense of humor, there are other ways to create a positive reframe.

Positive Reframing

Ask yourself if there's anything of value in your situation. There's usually something, no matter how negative the situation seems. In the cubicle life, you're getting a pay-check. When the computer is unresponsive, you might still get Twitter or solitaire. The cat *is* cute.

During sleepless nights, you can brainstorm a list of positive values—in your mind, with a pen, or using finger puppets. This allows your reframe to have new plot twists rather than the well-worn negative one.

Think of making a positive reframe like taking a piece of art to a frame shop. The wrong color matte or frame can wash the artwork out or make it look chintzy, but the right color can make even a magazine ad look classy. Same thing is true when you shop for the scarf or shirt to make you look soft and gorgeous, or dashing and classy.

This time, you're reframing the picture of your life—both the days and the sleepless nights.

Reframe Insomnia

Once when I explained Restful Insomnia to a new acquaintance, she replied in a soft drawl, "Isn't insomnia great? I just love that time of night. In fact, when I sleep right through the night, I miss it."

All of you who agree with her, please raise your hands. Hmmm . . . I see four of you with hands partway up. The rest of you million readers (a little positive image for the author here) spend sleepless nights being worried, grumpy, and wanting to sleep already.

That was me last night, when I hadn't had insomnia in a while. I was roused awake by my son thumping through the house. After yelling at him to stop (I was too tired to get out of bed), I started wondering if I should just get up and write this chapter, although my body could barely make it to bed five minutes before. *Grump, grump, grump, I'll never get back to sleep, I'm not feeling well, I should write, I should sleep, how could he do that to me?*

Then I remembered Restful Insomnia. I didn't have to be this grumpy; I could change what I told myself. My mantra became *It's OK to just rest . . . put on the eye mask and roll your eyes down . . . breathe . . .* And indeed, Restful Insomnia worked—once I let it. I became rested, so it didn't matter if I slept (and I did).

Although I've had several years of practice reframing insomnia, you can make a difference in your view of wakefulness in just one night.

Sleep Beliefs

The first step is to be aware of who you are when you're awake at night. What beliefs do you have about insomnia and sleep?

- Is sleep your paragon of happiness—nothing else will do?
- Is slumber something you disdain for "lesser" beings?
- Do you run through the insomnia cures, furious that you're awake?
- Are you afraid of sleep, of lowering your guard on emotions or household security?
- Do you think sleep wastes your time, keeping you from matching the productivity of your sleepless boss?
- Do you worry that each second of sleep you miss will make you less healthy and productive?
- Do you think sleep will come once you solve the world's problems (or at least your personal problems)?

While you'd rather sleep—or at least your body would—your beliefs may push for you to check e-mail, triple-check the doors, watch the clock to see if you're asleep yet, or sit up and listen for every noise. Beliefs have a powerful hold on the mind and body, though they can be changed.

Reframing Insomnia
Step back from your beliefs and look at the sleepless time from a different perspective. Reframe insomnia by finding something valuable about the time at night when you're awake—even one tiny thing that's agreeable to your body.

One of these ideas might spark you:

- Resting the body
- Reading
- Quieting the mind

- Being horizontal
- Digesting experiences and food from the day
- Making new connections
- Being dreamy and creative
- Writing
- Drawing
- Not talking
- Listening to your inner voice
- Befriending your body, or just being with it
- Meditating
- Breathing
- Practicing yoga
- Watching your sweetheart sleep

Gifts of Insomnia

I learned how to reframe insomnia from watching my husband, a man who could sleep in a carnival midway. If he was awakened, he turned over, closed his eyes, and calmly returned to sleep. From him I realized that the volume of irritation in my head was louder than the car waking me up as it raced down the street.

As my body imitated what he did, my mind picked up some calm traits as well. I learned that insomnia can be a weird and wonderful gift.

What's the gift for you? It might be in what insomnia is teaching you: that you need exercise, take medications that don't work together, drink too much caffeine, or have emotions that want attention.

It might be the gift of time to pay attention to yourself. You have time to heal, restore, and relax, just like you wish you had during the day. OK, it's a little later than planned, but it's a gift you can accept.

While it's easy to spend night-years in stress (worrying about things not getting done, being furious at your dog's snoring, or being angry at yourself for being too worried to sleep), you can take back your nightlife while you can't sleep. Do this by focusing on the gifts: read a novel, deepen your intuition, or heal your physical and emotional self with mysterious nighttime energy.

Using insomnia is in your hands. Put your body at the helm, and go on an unexpectedly fruitful trip. This book is your travel guide on the journey.

Chapter 4

Creating a Night Nest

*Is there a more gentle way to go into the night /
than to follow an endless rope of sentences /
and then to slip drowsily under the surface of a page . . .*
—Billy Collins, poet

ON A COTTAGE PORCH I SAW A NEST—a mess of brown feathers and twigs and shards of blue eggshells. I thought it was abandoned until I touched it and baby robins perked up, flapped their little wings, and opened their huge yellow beaks. After they realized I wasn't a mama bird with food, they snuggled back into their nest. They had a safe place to wait, to nurture, and to grow until they learned to fly and pick their own worms.

You also need a safe place to wait, to nurture, to grow, to renew until sleep returns with its dream morsels. You need a Night Nest.

Your Night Nest creates an environment to soothe your insomnia. Without it—when your night environment stimulates your eyes, movement, or thoughts—you don't deeply rest. Instead, you're engaged in a battle: the body is exhausted, yet the mind wants to be productive. Neither side wins.

You can create a supportive night environment where both your tired body and mind can rest. Your Night Nest sets the stage for peace, renewal, and inner creativity.

Erica liked her bedroom during the day—moss green walls, leaf-pattern bedspread, watercolor paintings on the walls. (She redecorated after her divorce.) But she hated her room in the middle of the night. She woke around 3 A.M. to the orangish city lights, the menacing shadows by the door, the twist of the quilt hot on her skin. Her face glowed, her nightgown clung between her breasts, and her thoughts ran high. Insomnia plus a hot flash—exhausted, sweaty, and awake.

Erica smoothed her sheets, turned her pillow to the cooler side, and extended an arm and leg outside the quilt as a body thermostat. Breathe . . . rest . . . breathe . . . rest . . . damn. Too hot, too hot. *What about the marketing presentation due next week? What about that scum my daughter's dating? What about the ivy taking over the side fence? I need to pee.*

Erica squinted as she turned on the lamp and walked the lit hall to the bathroom. She straightened some towels, peed, checked idly for new wrinkles, rinsed her face and neck, clipped a hangnail, retraced the steps to her bedroom, and changed into a dry nightgown. Then she shuffled downstairs to turn off the dining room light her daughter had left on, put some bowls in the dishwasher, trudged back upstairs, opened a window, and wriggled into bed. *I just want to sleep.*

Only she was awake. And tomorrow would be hell. Might as well read that quarterly sales account for marketing.

She leaned against the maple headboard, pushed her dark hair behind her ears, and waded through sales figures and analysis. The alarm clock changed its square numbers from 3:16 to 4:05 to 4:32. *Concentrate, Erica, or you'll have to read this report again tomorrow . . . after a latte or two.* Her eyes and body drooped. She felt cool again, and cuddled under the quilt. *Maybe I can get an hour and a half of sleep before the alarm.* The room was dark, her body was still, but her mind wouldn't turn off. *Damn.*

When Erica came to talk about her sleeplessness, I explained that she moved into a daytime mode during her insomnia. When she turned on the lights and did daytime activities (cleaning and working), Erica activated her Conscious Mind. The Conscious Mind likes to *do* things. It stimulates the body and thoughts to keep up with its *doing* quest.

Erica needed to create an environment to soothe her body and Conscious Mind. Then she could stay cozy with the Unconscious Mind a little longer, helping her renew even if she was not actually asleep.

Your Night Nest

The Night Nest provides comfort so your Unconscious Mind can expand its creative, healing, and restorative self. Your Night Nest has two parts: the environment of your room, and specific comfort items in your nest or stash.

Start by changing your environment to reduce distractions and irritations so "shoulds" don't creep into your insomnia. Before going to bed, straighten the piles of papers and clothes monsters on the floor; smooth your sheets so you don't wrestle with bed ogres; darken your windows; remove objects that create disconcerting shadows. If you move to another room so you don't wake your partner, create a soothing place there. Or do some Feng Shui.

Intuitive Feng Shui

Feng shui is the ancient Asian art of changing the energy flow in structures and rooms. It's done through arranging furniture, mirrors—even doors, windows, and the placement of structures on a property. I became intrigued with what I call Intuitive Feng Shui during chronic insomnia. I imagined how gentle, inviting energy would flow through the room, which engaged my Unconscious Mind and connected me in a very loving way to my bedroom. Later on I studied feng shui (I like the book *Sacred Space* by Denise Linn), but I still prefer to continue using my intuition during the night hours.

Envision the energy of light and air moving through your space. Does it come in from the window or door? Does it get stuck and swirl in nooks? Does it blow right through from window to door, like a wind in a wind tunnel cleaning everything out? Or does it feel like there's no fresh energy coming in at all?

Suzie played with feng shui at night. She realized in my class that she'd started having real trouble sleeping when she moved into a basement apartment. It had high windows, a door at the top of the stairs, and was full of clutter. She was overwhelmed trying to figure out how to get the time and money to fix the rental—and sleep or rest. I reminded her that she had influence on the energy in her room as well as the physical space. For a few nights, she imagined changing the flow of energy, sending it to the nook where her bed was located. Then during the day she opened the shades, straightened some of the mess, and put up small mirrors to reflect energy from the windows into the corners of the room. Eventually, she brought in plants to support the energy flow the room needed. She created a space for herself at night with energy that moved in ways that felt right.

Then Suzie put what she needed for the night by her bed.

Everything You Need at Hand

Create a soothing stash of items to ease your eyes, ears, body, and heart—this is your Night Nest. I've created mine over years of insomnia. It helps the body stay calm, so you don't trigger the mind during insomnia.

My Night Nest stays under my bed. It's in a blue-and-white flowered hatbox my mother sent me decades ago. It's filled with nighttime goodies—a buckwheat bolster for tight back muscles, lip balm, a water bottle to moisten my mouth, dim book lights, tissues. Nearby, I keep a white-noise machine to distance the barking dog. Everything is at my fingers so I don't have to gallivant through the house to find what I need.

Make your own Night Nest to keep close at hand while you're awake at night. Place your items in a shoe box under your bed, in a drawer in your nightstand, or in a knitter's bag or basket. Locate your Night Nest so you can reach it easily in your own bed or (if you journey to another room so as not to disturb your mate) near your comfort spot. Here's a tip: store it out of sight during the day, so it will remind you of the night when you use it.

Use the list that follows and your imagination to create a personalized "night spa" for your sleepless hours. (Many items for your Night Nest are available on the Restful Insomnia Web site or other sites listed in the resource section at the end of the book.) Start with what soothes your body, and end with what sparks your dreams.

Basic comfort: Keep your comfort goodies nearby. That way you won't be triggered about work as you pass by your briefcase looking for what you need.

- Hand lotion. Rough hands create irritation.
- Lip balm. It keeps me from licking my lips and relaxes the jaw.
- A water bottle. It gets rid of that sleepy cotton mouth.
- Tissues.
- Saline nasal spray for a stuffy nose.
- Over-the-counter medicines like Advil or Tylenol for head and body aches.
- Cough drops. (Even a little tickling cough keeps me from resting.)
- Massage oil or a shoulder massager.
- A washcloth or T-shirt if you get hot at night. You might try black cohosh tablets for menopausal night flashes (if your doctor agrees first).
- Bach Flower Rescue remedy or Calms Forté to calm the nerves. These homeopathic remedies have minuscule doses—they may act as a placebo, but they work for me.

Soft light: If you need light to write, read, or adjust your covers, use *low* light. Darkness stimulates your pituitary gland to produce the sleep hormone melatonin. Your mind stays dreamier in soft light.

> **Book light.** Book lights illuminate the page of your book or writing pad. Some clip to the back of your book: think of retractable flashlights. Or they hang around your neck. Others have a wedge of red lights that keep your eyes adjusted for low light—similar

to what the U.S. Coast Guard uses for night maneuvers. Another kind covers your reading page with a lit acrylic sheet. If you use book lights often, store extra batteries in your Night Nest.

Night pen. Night pens have lights in the shaft to illuminate the page, so you can see your scrawl after a nightly inspiration. Avoid those with harsh lights.

Flashlight lantern. Some camping flashlights open to become soft lantern lights. They illuminate a larger area than the book light and work well with regular pens.

Lamp scarf. A scarf dims the lamp by the bed when you need a little more lighting than you can get with a book light or a night pen. Drape the scarf around the lamp shade. (Stupidity warning: I almost burned a scarf once by putting it over the top of the lightbulb.) Some people use a lamp dimmer—though many dimmers emit a faint whine when the light's on low.

Writing and reading: Reading or writing can agitate you or pacify you, depending on the topic. A pen and paper in your Night Nest help you note an interesting dream, great idea, or to-do list that won't let go.

Pens. Even though I have a night pen, I use regular pens before lights-out or when I use a lantern light. Black ink shows up better in soft light. Red ink is hard to see in dim light.

Notebook. A notebook is easy to grab and maps your Restful Insomnia journey. Stick a Post-it tab on the clean sheet so you won't write over earlier scribblings, if you choose to keep lights off.

Books and magazines. Comforting books and magazines help your Unconscious Mind lead; your Conscious Mind follows someone else's images. Stash some favorites: the *New Yorker* or *O* magazine; favorite children's books (*Charlotte's Web*); books with short sections (Jack Kornfield's *Buddha's Little Instruction Book*); humor (Bailey White's *Mama Makes Up Her Mind*); poetry (Garrison Keillor's *Good Poems*); hypnotic books (Ragini Michaels's *Facticity*); spiritual readings (Sharon Salzberg's *Faith*); gardening (Marianne Binetti's *Easy Answers for Great Gardens*); old mystery or romantic favorites that you can put down when you feel drowsy—because you know how they turn out.

Soothers: Let your body sink into a soothing aura of sounds, darkness, and comfort.

Eye mask. Good eye masks make a soothing, dark difference when the city lights flicker, someone leaves the hall light on, or your eyes feel extrasensitive to light. Little satin ones from pharmacies get steamy and shift on the face. Bucky's eye masks use polar fleece, a foam roll to keep light from peeping in the bottom, and adjustable elastic Velcro straps. The darkness and soft pressure remind your body of deep sleep or rest at night—especially during the summer light.

White noise. White noise is a "sssshhh" sound, just like from a fan. White noise (a broad audio-frequency range) diminishes the intensity of individual sounds. As I mentioned earlier, think of noise like a picture: a dog barking when you're asleep sounds sharp— like the contrast of a black silhouette on white paper. White noise makes the background gray, so the noise stands out less.

White noise comes from running a fan, switching on a sleep machine, or playing a special alarm clock that plays digitally recorded sounds of rain, waves, or wind. (I don't like the repeat loop on digital recordings— I'm an audio-neurotic and it bugs me to hear the exact same seagull call every two minutes.) You can play CDs of ocean waves, Oregon rivers, Hawaiian waterfalls, beaches, or rainstorms. There are even recordings of vacuum cleaners, air conditioners, and clothes dryers.

Babies like white noise because it sounds like they're still inside the uterus with sounds of their mother's heartbeat, breathing, and blood flow. You remember that, don't you? Even if you don't, the sound still can soothe the Unconscious Mind.

Earplugs. Some people love the inner quiet of earplugs—like being in a silent cocoon. Earplugs remind you to stop attending to interruptions. The best earplugs for sleeping fit in the ear canal, remain soft, and stay in place while you move in the night. They're made from lots of materials: natural rubber, silicone, wax and cotton, plastic, polyurethane, or PVC foam. And they come in lots of shapes: tubes that expand in your ear canal, preformed ovals that slide in, cubes to mold and flatten (like Silly Putty), half-dome inserts with mini-plastic grips, hollow plastic teardrops attached to cords. They're not expensive in small quantities, so check out a few to see how they work for you.

Relaxation CDs. Hypnotic or relaxation CDs help you follow your Unconscious Mind. Preview CDs before you buy them at certain stores or at the library.

Music. Music affects your heartbeat, breathing rate, pulse, blood pressure, and limbic system—your "emotional brain." To rest at night, use relaxing slow music with a regular tempo—your heart aligns to the beat. Try out instrumental music (no words to stimulate you), songs in an unfamiliar language, or spiritual or meditational music with repetitive chants. My favorite is Tibetan gongs.

Aromatherapy. A soothing smell can alter your state of mind. Use an aromatherapy kit to heat scented oils, or place drops of them on a cotton ball. Try chamomile, rose, lavender, or marjoram. Spritz perfume or scented water (for example, rose water). Or keep herbs—lavender, thyme, rosemary, lemon balm, hyssop—in an airtight container, to open and smell when the occasion arises.

Sexual aids. Sexual pleasure can take the tension out of your body. (Although for a few, it jazzes rather than relaxes insomnia.) Certain playthings make being in bed feel more relaxed and pleasurable. You can buy a lubricant, vibrator, or other gadgets at a positive sex store like the Babeland Web site.

Bolster pillow. If your body feels tense or numb, a neck-roll pillow or rolled towel can aid in muscle release. Prop up your crunched shoulders, neck, or lower back as you rest or stretch in Night Yoga. A small bolster pillow filled with buckwheat hulls provides continued support without sagging.

Special talismans and trinkets. Find items to remind yourself of tranquility at night—tranquility in your real life and in your imagined world. What speaks to your heart? A stone from the shores of Lake Erie, a corner of your baby blanket, a polished purple amethyst, a love note from courtship, a photo of you relaxing at the beach, the charm bracelet your grandmother wore, a birthday poem from your daughter, a picture of your dream vacation in Italy, a snapshot of your grandson, a quote from a spiritual leader, affirmations of your success? . . . Your talismans tell your body that you are loved—a sensation that makes it easier to relax.

The sensation of insomnia became calmer for Erica once she began using her Night Nest. When she awoke hot and groggy, she reached for her towel, wiped off her face and neck, then rested in dreamy half sleep a while longer. Erica relied on night-lights to walk safely to the bathroom. She appreciated her body instead of looking for wrinkles in the mirror. Back in her room, she straightened her covers, sipped from her water bottle, and slipped back into bed. She propped the bolster pillow under her spine, letting her chest open after a day huddled over the computer. She felt her muscles let go, her breathing deepen. When her mind started racing over work, she turned on the book light and wrote her best solutions in her journal. If thoughts of her daughter's boyfriend intruded—*Can't change that tonight.* Erica opened *House and Garden* magazine and visualized a remodeled kitchen. Her eyes grew tired. She switched the book light off. She cuddled and drifted in and out of drowsiness. Sleep finally returned. Her Night Nest led her to soothe the wakeful hours.

Chapter 5

Evening Rituals

I had this whole ritual with my mother making the bed
with me inside it so I would be invisible.
—Ahmet Zappa, musician

RITUALS IN THE MORNING, during mealtimes, on the
Fourth of July, on birthdays, at funerals—even TGIF
(Thank God It's Friday)—create structure, routine,
and rhythm in your life. Rituals wake you up, remind
you to eat and move, provide celebration, allow you to
grieve, and connect you to the sun, moon, and revo-
lution of the earth. Evening Rituals guide you as day
changes to night.

Centuries ago, rituals were automatic when the sun set (it's hard to do the laundry in the dark). Now, with bright cities and homes, we need to use our habits to create our transitions.

Daniel dozed during his 7:30 A.M. English class. He had fallen asleep at 2 A.M. the night before—early for him. "My teacher yells at me because I can't stay awake," he sighed, pushing his blond bangs out of his eyes. "I guess I could go to sleep earlier, but I can't wind down."

Daniel sprawled on the blue carpet in the family room, adjusting a couch pillow under his neck. His weary parents listened from the breakfast nook. His mom felt worn out by Daniel's erratic nights and sleepy days. She knew that teens often have later bedtimes and rising times, but Daniel's were worse than normal. He hadn't gotten much better after his treatment for mild sleep apnea and ADHD (attention deficit/hyperactivity disorder). Maybe Restful Insomnia would help him—and the family—regain some sanity.

Daniel's chaotic sleep patterns started with his jam-packed and zoned-out evenings. After dinner, Daniel sprawled on his bed (the center of his nonparent universe) and did homework, watched TV, listened to music, hung out with friends, played video games, texted or Twittered on the cell phone, checked Facebook on his laptop, played guitar.

And occasionally slept.

"My parents and brothers go to bed around eleven or twelve," he said. "I know I'll feel trashed in school if I stay up, but I'm just not tired." He couldn't order himself to sleep. "I crash later," he explained—"On top of the covers with the TV still on," added his dad, who struggled to wake him in the mornings.

It's not just teens who live jam-packed lives. Evenings clamor with errands, housework, laundry, dishes, checking e-mail, helping with homework, making phone calls, working until the body collapses.

Perhaps you zone out for a break—talk with a friend, play computer games, watch television shows. Your body lies on the couch while your mind is stimulated by lights, stories, emotions (TV shows go for sadness and excitement)—the day's still with you.

Zoned-out or crammed evenings don't lead to rest and sleep. But Evening Rituals turn the *doing* day into a *being* night.

The Rhythm of Cycles

Evening Rituals are not another five-minute task to add to the hundreds of five-minute tasks in your day. (I keep thinking that if we added all the five-minute tasks together, we wouldn't have time to eat.) Evening Rituals are not religious, not formal, not detailed obsessive-compulsive procedures (like, say, putting perfect hospital corners on your sheets). Evening Rituals don't come from your overloaded mind. Instead, your body guides you from day to night.

Evening Rituals help you:

- Relax into your body (and remember that you have one)
- Remind your body to soothe itself, even when your mind is racing
- Let your Unconscious Mind set the stage for sleep, rest, and Restful Insomnia

Let's start by understanding the opposite of Evening Rituals.

From Doing to Being

Morning Rituals bring on your day. They help your mind and body communicate so you can transition from *being* to *doing*. Morning Rituals moor your Unconscious Mind on its night raft and let your Conscious Mind take the lead.

Evening Rituals do the opposite. They park your Conscious Mind and loosen your Unconscious Mind on the night raft. They take you from *doing* to *being*.

Evening Rituals release the day—work, errands, friends, homework, bills, dirty laundry.

I bet you grew up with an Evening Ritual. Babies have particular routines for bed: cuddling a stuffed dog or blanket, nursing or a bottle, clean clothes, songs, a darkened room, a kiss on the cheek, a pat on the back, and *good night.* Bedtime habits, say parenting experts, teach babies and young children that night is for sleep and rest.

We need Evening Rituals as adults as much as ever. That is, we need to make our evening routines (brushing teeth, taking vitamins, kissing loved ones good night) more than habits. When we deepen these routines with an awareness that we're moving toward rest, we create a path to let go of our busy minds.

My sister has precise Evening Rituals. The bed is made up tightly in flannel sheets, her teeth are brushed with an electric toothbrush, and she reads a chapter in a mystery book.

My mother has her own routines. She phones friends, cleans the kitchen, plays solitaire on the computer, and watches television until the redecorating show makes her yawn. She says that her evenings mellow her out, though she has trouble winding down or turning the lights off before midnight. Within her unmoving body churns an active mind.

Zoning Out Doesn't Mellow You Out

A Japanese study of computer users and sleep found that when subjects used the Internet—especially playing computer games—over half had delayed bedtimes and shortened sleeping hours. Lack of sleep, the researchers theorized, was due to shifting bright computer lights as well as the tension of computer games in the evenings. Television can have a similar effect.

Forget it, you grumble. *I need my TV to chill after a long day.* And you do need a break.

Television and computers send tension to the background with a flick of the switch or the mouse. Good-bye to the mean boss, the shrinking checkbook balance, and the guy who hasn't phoned. Hello to friendly faces, laughter, car chases, clever blogs, politicians, celebrities, family rooms to be remodeled, murders to be solved. Your worries return? Turn on one more show, visit one more Web site, read one more blog, play one more game. Or make one more phone call.

Distracting your mind gives you a break, but not deep rest.

Finding Yourself in New Pleasures

Sarah moved to New York for a magazine job, though she hated to leave the Midwest. A graphic artist, she spent her evenings talking to or messaging her boyfriend and friends in Chicago about grad school, romances, concerts, and art shows. Bedtime got later and later. "I don't feel sleepy until about an hour or two after we're done," she said. "But I miss my friends." She also began to miss her sleep.

We worked together so Sarah could create time for her transitions at night.

Learning to say good night to the telephone (or the television and computer) is a two-part process. The first part creates limits; the second part connects you to other pleasures.

Sarah started by hanging up a few minutes earlier and earlier, until she hung up an hour before bed. She also turned the phone ringer off. TV junkies (that's me) can move the set, especially out of the bedroom. Turn down the sound or contrast. Television timers create automatic limits. Or put on a video of a fire in a hearth. For computers, use software programs to limit access. I created an alarm in my calendar program telling me to turn off the computer at ten each night. OK, I turn it off around ten-thirty, but I've stopped surfing until midnight.

Don't forget the power of your mind and decisions. Make an agreement with yourself or a friend to turn the electronics off and support the rhythms of your body.

Add new pleasures to fill in the void as you change your habits. Otherwise you'll substitute a brand-new habit (eating, smoking, drinking) or turn on *Brady Bunch* reruns.

Ask your body what it wants. If you feel lonely, listen to songs, play books on tape, or turn on the radio. One client put up pictures of friends and family for companionship. Magazines, new books, or old favorite novels provide easy reading (which helps your Conscious Mind let go). Moving the body or the hands provides creative freedom and quiet meditation. Some clients knit, learn to play the ukulele, or play solitaire with real cards (shuffle and deal them yourself—without a redeal).

Sarah wrote in her journal and crafted cards for friends. She connected to her artistic self in her Evening Rituals.

Creating Rituals

You already have habits that move you toward the night. Turn them into Evening Rituals by becoming aware of how they comfort your body and help you make the transition from day to night.

My clients have used the following techniques to soothe their evenings. If they practice new ideas for twenty-one days, they create a habit for bed.

Create a habit tonight.

Connect to Movement
- Exhale all the air out of your chest. A-l-l-l-l-l-l the air. It releases the day's stress.
- Take a deep breath. Expand your ribs into the tight spots behind your shoulders. Settle into your body with a steady flow of a few breaths.
- Raise your arms to the ceiling, then out to your sides. Slowly twist to the left and the right as you inhale and exhale.
- Take a night stroll around your yard or around the block, and experience the night.

Decrease the Buzz
- Darken and quiet your house in rooms you rarely use at night; turn off lights and appliances to settle into a serene environment.

- Lower the volume on the television, radio, or stereo.
- Relax with some evening music. Slower, soft music calms you. (As I mentioned in chapter 4, it decreases your heart rate, blood pressure, respiration rate, muscular tension, motor responses, and skin temperature.) Instrumental music keeps your mind from thinking about the lyrics. Unwind with a collection of adult lullabies.

Prepare Your House
- Close the blinds—it dims the streetlights reflecting through the windows.
- Straighten a room or corner so you have a place not filled with the day's mess.
- Do a few morning tasks (put out clean breakfast dishes, lunch containers, and ground beans for coffee) to have less to worry about at night. Choose clothes for the morning, and place the briefcase by the door.
- Lock (or double-check) doors and windows if you're a night worrier. Do you forget whether you've locked the doors or turned off the stove? I remind myself by saying loudly, "I, Sondra, am locking the front door" to set the task in my memory.
- Just like a child, you can say *good night* to your house—or simply appreciate it.

Turn Down the Voltage
- Dim the overhead lights and turn on a lamp. You'll increase the release of melatonin from your pineal gland as your home darkens.

- Reduce the electrical buzz in your house by turning off the television, computer (especially the monitor), VCR, lights, and Game Boys. I'm often not aware when the computer's on, though I do notice that the room feels calmer when it's off.
- Turn off "vampire" appliances—the ones that remain on standby, waiting for instant turn-on (many TV sets), or chargers that remain on after recharging batteries. You may feel a release when they're off for the night. (It's also good for the environment and your energy bill.)

Prepare Your Body

- Relax your body as you do your routine tasks: Stretch as you change into your PJs. Massage your cheeks as you rub cream on your face. Brush or run your fingers through your hair to shake off the day.
- Appreciate your body—even the parts that you wish were different—for how it functions.
- Use special treats to honor the evening. Bathe with Epsom salts or aromatherapy oils. Give yourself a foot massage with cream or vegetable oil (and wear socks to bed). Do some Night Yoga, like putting your feet up the wall. See other restorative moves in chapter 10, "Resting with Meditation."

Prepare Your Room

- Bring in some fresh water, and some books or magazines you'd like to read.
- Light a lamp; set the alarm. Open a window for fresh air at night.

Restful Insomnia

- Play some soft evening music.
- Turn down the sheets if you've made your bed. Or if you like your bed to "air" during the day (research shows that this reduces dust mites), smooth the sheets and blankets, and fluff the pillows.
- Straighten what's in front of your bed to have fewer distractions in the middle of the night. Put away your clothes; tidy that pile of papers.
- Spray a mist of rose water to clear the air, or warm some aromatherapy oils. Lavender, chamomile, neroli, rose, and marjoram are all very soothing.

Put Yourself to Bed
- Remember how great your own bed feels after a long vacation? Let your bed welcome you each night.
- If you're not ready to give up the television (melatonin or not), cuddle up in a favorite blanket, turn the volume down, and watch something soothing—a show, a video, or something easy to turn off. Don't watch the news— it's *designed* to keep you up.
- Read—it shifts you to a night mind. Your Conscious Mind follows a writer's images and stories; then it's ready to follow your Unconscious Mind for the night.
- If your mind ruminates over a busy tomorrow, write down what you'd like to do. Then put it aside.
- Write statements of gratitude—for anything that has brought you happiness or has taught you something today, or during your life.
- Connect with a power greater than your mind—the universe, your Essence, a Higher Power, God . . .

whatever name you use. Pray or give thanks for where you've been. Asking for help lets you remember that you have resources beyond what you imagine.

- Write what you'd like to dream about. Many "dream watchers" discover that what they write is what appears in their dreams.
- Write down what you'd like to learn, heal, or let go of during the night.
- Breathe deeply. Feel the safety of your house—or create invisible guardians around it.

Put Yourself to Rest—and Perhaps Sleep

- Notice how the darkness in your room provides space for imagination and rest.
- Feel your body within your sheets, under your blankets, and next to your pillows. Your house, room, and bed all cushion you.
- Say hello to the night. Imagine how your body will rest, how you will follow the Unconscious Mind, and how you will feel renewed.

Daniel's Evening Ritual

We found ways to give Daniel's room a sleepier, more relaxed feel in the evenings—even while his TV and/or computer were going. He turned off the overhead light and turned on his nightstand lamp. He considered turning off the television and listening to music—at least on Wednesdays, when he was bored with what was on. He liked NightYoga, especially the pose where he'd lie on his back with his feet up the wall. He could do it in bed. His noise machine helped him sleep, so he'd switch it on low when his parents went to bed.

He needed a small ritual he could do each night to help trigger his Unconscious Mind into a sleepier mode. Maybe he had that trigger when he was a boy. I asked, "What was your bedtime like when you were little?"

His mother piped up: "He wouldn't go to bed without his favorite quilt. He took it to sleepovers until he was eleven."

"Yeah, my airplane quilt," added Daniel, a bit sheepishly. "I picked out the fabric. I still have it on a chair in my room."

Could he use it now as part of his Evening Ritual? "Spread it on your bed or straighten it out," I suggested. "That way, you'll remember that your bed is meant for sleep."

Daniel nodded. "I still like that quilt."

A month later, I talked to Daniel's mother to see if his Evening Ritual ideas had taken hold.

"He's still Daniel," she said, "but the television was on fewer mornings when his dad woke him up, and the blanket was spread on the bed." Some nights when his mom went to bed late, Daniel's lights were low and the television off. It was a start.

Daniel's Evening Ritual introduced him to making friends with the night. Like most good friendships, relationships take time to build.

Chapter 6

Getting into Your Body

Without the body, the wisdom of
the larger self cannot be known.
—John Conger

LORETTA WAS SMART—she'd finish the Saturday *New York Times* crossword puzzle before lunch. But her smarts were all in her mind. The only time she really experienced her body was when she had no other choice: running a marathon, having intense sex, being sick. Other times, it was as if her body used sign language . . . and she was blind.

"I'm angry," she said one day when she came in for coaching.

"How do you know you're angry?" I asked. Loretta looked surprised.

"Well, I keep having this argument in my head with my husband, where he's not listening to me."

"And how do you feel?"

"Feel? I feel angry!" she snapped.

"What does anger feel like in your body?"

"Um . . . I don't know. I guess I feel tense," she answered.

"Where in your body do you feel tense?"

Loretta looked perplexed, closed her eyes, then said, "I think my stomach."

"Good. That's the sensation of anger for you right now. And it will change over time."

In Restful Insomnia you want to let go of your mind to rest, but where do you go? Your body. Rather than rushing through sensations—anger, hunger, sleepiness, illness— to decide what to *do* about them, you descend and experience your body. Then your body has room for its natural process of rest and healing. However, many insomniacs don't know how to let go.

Loretta knew her body as if it was a Google map rather than a place. She could see that Mealtime Avenue crossed Anger Boulevard and Tired Street. But she had no idea about the bumps in the roads or the scenery along the way.

This chapter discusses ways you can experience your body—its energy, emotions, illness, tension, relaxation, and rest.

Awareness 101

Where are your hands right now? Are they touching the book, holding a mug of coffee, tucked under the blankets on your bed? Notice what one hand experiences: the edges of the paper, steam of the latte, or texture of the wool.

Move your focus to your foot. Do you feel the shoe or the sheet? Focus on your legs, back, even your lips and eyes.

You're moving your attention to the sensations on the outside of your body. You can move this attention inwardly as well. Start with your breath. Can you feel air moving through your nostrils, letting your lungs expand, then contract? How about your digestive system—your throat, stomach, intestines? Can you become aware of the sensations in your heart, feeling the beat?

It's common to notice the heart for a moment, then wander off to consider whether coffee makes your heart beat faster. We're so used to thinking in this culture; it takes a little practice and repetition to come back to the sensations. Not only do sensations change; they pave roadways of body wisdom.

Awareness 201

To go deeper into your awareness of sensations, allow yourself to first notice the physically "real" sensations, such as texture, warmth, and tension. Then experiment if you have an intuition or imagination of an inner sensation: color, vibration, or tone.

Remember your body knows more than your mind, a difficult realization for those with strong minds. If you try to impose a sensation, say a color on your stomach (*It's green; I've eaten a salad, so it's green*), it can work for a moment. But if your mind spaces out or you keep getting a different sensation, your body's telling you it needs to follow its own wisdom. Try imagining being deep inside your stomach instead of watching it from your head. What sounds are inside, what do you see, do you feel heat or movement? *The food is green, and the digestive energy is a wave of red.*

There is no right answer to what you notice. Your body changes, your ability to perceive your body changes, and each connection provides information on who you are right now. If there are waves of red energy in the digestion, they might evoke the anger you've had since your sweetie—ex-sweetie—broke up with you. If you're holding that resentment in your stomach, it could explain why you can't eat much more than salads lately. Especially when you think about how you were lied to.

Thoughts and Emotions

You're probably aware that sensations come from the smell of a rose, the tingle of salsa, or the tension from sitting over a computer. Did you know that sensations also come from thoughts, most clearly when those thoughts have emotional content? Many people, like Loretta, are surprised to realize that emotions cause a physical reaction.

When we were working together, Loretta paged through various thoughts to notice her physical reaction. *I have to get eggs at the store*—not much reaction. *I wish my friend Fred hadn't moved to Ohio*—long exhales and a little teariness. *My husband is talking about those multiplayer computer games again*—strong exhales and tightness in her stomach.

She kept focused on her body: her shoulders were pulled up and there was a kind of heat, red and orange flames. . . . Oh yes, anger. *How could he even think about those again? Didn't he remember how he played them all night until I almost left? I need to talk to him NOW about not playing again.* Return to the body: the fire in her stomach, hands, jaw, and brow. It almost felt like too much until she tapped her acupressure points with Energy Psychology. (See chapter 11, "Emotions and Touch.")

As she stayed with the sensations, the flames turned to a wobbly feeling—bluish and kind of cold. She sighed, like letting air and tension out. Tears came, and awareness of the stress they both were under with their jobs. Sure, he was thinking about games, but she had spent more time shopping.

She could change something in herself to connect with him, not just get mad. She wasn't sure what to do yet, but maybe it would come as she rested in the night. Her awareness of her body and emotions changed her thinking, so she had more options.

Dialogue

When I first started working with my body, my mind made me very confused. I couldn't tell if I was feeling a sensation, or if I was thinking about a sensation I thought I should feel; *Am I really feeling gray vibrations in my chest, or do I just think I should cry?* If you're like this, try having a dialogue between your body and your Conscious Mind.

The first step is to separate the two, so you know the difference between the experience of your body and the experience of your Conscious Mind.

- Imagine you can hold your Conscious Mind in one hand and your body in the other.
- Give wherever you have the strongest body sensations—your stomach, your fingers, the back of your neck—a mystical mouth to speak with. That's your body. Then notice the parts that seem to hold your thoughts (your brain, feet, jaw). Give that—the mouth or even your Conscious Mind—a computer printout.
- Lean to one side as you experience your Conscious Mind and to the other side as you experience your body.

Now that you've separated your Conscious Mind and body, you need to find out if they're willing to have a conversation with each other—or to share with you. If not, perhaps a part needs help—it could come as reassurance, a Spiritual Center translator, or acceptance. Still "no"? Try again in a few minutes, or use the writing technique described later in this chapter.

To have the dialogue, start by having the Conscious Mind ask any body part what it wants to say. Maybe that body part is afraid of something, or needs something from the Conscious Mind, or just wants to do whatever the heck it wants, without criticism.

Then reverse, and see if the body has questions for the Conscious Mind, such as why it keeps criticizing, why it always has a list of things to do, or the questions in the "Writing or Drawing" section that follows.

As the body and Conscious Mind listen to each other, you may discover some old patterns, and new ways of relating. Even small changes can make a big difference over time.

Writing or Drawing

Perhaps you'd like to write or draw the dialogue between the Conscious Mind and the body. During insomnia, keep the lighting dim. (The process is more important than a perfect product.) Use a different body position—or even a different hand—for each side. If you're writing or drawing, ask some of the following questions:

- What's the strongest sensation? What's the Conscious Mind reaction to that sensation?
- What's the biggest fear?
- How does the body or Conscious Mind appear when the fear is gone?
- How does the body relate to the Conscious Mind, and vice versa?

As you deepen the communication between the body and Conscious Mind, in whatever form, the relationship provides wisdom you can take into your days.

Humming and Stretching

I started humming in Restful Insomnia after a yoga class, where we said a few "oms" as we sat in a meditation. I'd never chanted before—it had always seemed too much in the realm of monks in orange robes. But I liked it. It kept my mind from wandering as much: I noticed my body and each breath.

Later, during a sleepless night, I thought of chanting to connect with my body. So I hummed with each exhale. Try it. *Hmmmmmmmmmmmmmmmm.* You can feel the vibrations in your lungs and throat, and you can hear the subtle sound coming from your nose. Send the hum around your body in your imagination. Are your shoulders tense? Let the vibration loosen the muscles. Do your feet feel numb? Let the hum enliven them.

To connect to your body at night, change the hum to reflect different energy. The excitement in the ribs might be *hm-hm-hm.* Sadness in the eyes could lower in pitch; tension in the neck might generate a grumble.

Humming works great with stretching, which was also inspired by that same yoga class. Stretching is more subtle than Night Yoga (see chapter 10), and easier to do without waking a bed partner. Expand the ribs with that *hm-hm-hm* to feel the excitement move. Scrunch or widen the eyes as you lower the pitch. Curl the neck as you grumble.

Humming and stretching are avenues of communication that allow you to become more familiar with the energy of your lovely body.

Restful Insomnia Body at Night

Loretta developed a routine to follow when her mind was going on its usual nightly race, with sleep far in the distance.

First, she had to remember she had a body. (That's a common problem for insomniacs, to get caught in the thoughts—the body is just a hat rack for the brain.) After re-adjusting her pillow, Loretta would let out a deep sigh that would remind her to use her body to rest.

Her Conscious Mind said, *Just ignore the body; you'll fall asleep as soon as we figure out these problems.*

She put her hands on her stomach. Touching made it easier to connect. She'd focus on her skin or breath.

Then she'd focus on the strongest sensation in her body—could be tension, relaxation, or an emotion. She'd stay with it for a few minutes, reminding herself to notice the senses—the colors or image, the sound (a tone or even a song), the sense of how it felt or vibrated. Even a taste or a smell.

Loretta followed the sensations as they changed, even subtly. Being in the body lowered the intensity of insomnia, giving the Conscious Mind a rest. Loretta found that her body was a lot smarter than she'd given it credit for.

Chapter 7

Night Yoga

Blessed are the flexible,
for they shall not be bent out of shape.
—Author unknown

AT SIX IN THE MORNING, my friend Michael started bak-
ing the best Italian cookies you could imagine: cannoli
with ricotta, anise-laced *imbragioni,* sesame Neapolitans.
He mixed twenty-pound bags of flour, ten-pound bags of
sugar, vats of lemon oil, and tins of butter. Then he pulled
dough from giant bowls to cut, shape, and bake. After
a day of running on the cement-floor kitchen, dashing
through the cooler, and standing in front of the hot oven,

his whole body was exhausted, though the boss and customers were happy.

Michael hit the sack at ten o'clock, but he couldn't wind down. His shoulders scrunched up to his neck, his legs ached from hips to toes, and it hurt him to open his hands. He just wanted to sleep, to let go of the customers who whined about anise instead of chocolate, the boss who wanted three dozen extra biscotti by noon, and the rude bus driver on the way home. Though he tried to relax, his body wouldn't let go.

I suggested that Night Yoga would help release both his body and his mind, especially on nights after he worked. Night Yoga consists of easy stretches to help the body release the tension of the day. I integrated these poses from my fourteen years of yoga practice. If people can do this ancient bodywork sitting at a desk instead of on a mat in a yoga studio, they can certainly do it in bed.

No, I didn't do Downward Dog on the bed. (Downward Dog is a yoga pose where your feet are on the floor, your butt is high in the air, and your hands are a few feet in front of your toes.) Instead, I settled into the night with gentle hip openers, yogic breathing called *pranayama,* chest openers, restorative poses, twists, and resting inversions. I've done Night Yoga mostly in bed, although some of my clients have done poses in a dimly lit room or on the floor—keeping warm and relaxed—and then moved back to bed, more relaxed in the body.

I've based these Night Yoga poses on my years of practice, supplemented by some great books and input by my teacher Irene Alexander.

Overview

It's important that your yoga time is restful. (Instead of reading while doing Night Yoga, you may want to tape yourself saying the instructions, so you can listen while you stretch.) But make sure you're gentle with yourself. These Night Yoga reminders can help you keep a slow and calm relationship with your body at night:

* Do these poses very gently.
* Breathe. Inhale softness and exhale tension.
* Pay attention to your body as you settle into your bones, gravity, and the night.
* No pain? Good. It's not a competition—not even a competition with yourself.

After each pose, breathe. Relax. Notice the sensations and rhythms in your body.

Props: In a yoga studio, it can take five minutes after class to put back the blocks, blankets, straps, wedges, and mats. While I don't suggest that pile of props for Night Yoga (use whatever you have on hand), consider including in your Night Nest an extra blanket or two for padding and to keep you warm and some buckwheat roll pillows. An eye pillow can relax your eyes while you're in a pose.

Night Yoga Poses

In these instructions, I lead you through breathing, twists, hip openers, and gentle inversions. Although you may do them on the floor or on the bed, I've used the word *bed* just to keep it simple.

Use the poses that allow you to feel opening and release—could be one favorite or all of them, depending on the night. Or use easier poses, to allow more rest. Listen to your body—it knows what it needs.

Breathing

Yoga practice is a great way to get reacquainted with your breath. These instructions cover some basic breathing exercises and alternate-nostril breathing (which, although it's a little odd, can really change your body patterns).

An important note from yoga instructor Irene Alexander: "Breathing practice can be extremely relaxing and helpful. And it is very common for people to have some feelings of anxiety that arise from even just watching the breath, but especially from lengthening the breath. If anxiety arises, just bring the breath back to a place and pace that are comfortable."

Start with breathing awareness, and move to other breathing practices if your body wants to. Remember, whatever your breathing pattern, be gentle and natural with it: befriend it, learn from it, and let it comfort you.

Breathing Awareness

Just notice your breath, without changing it too much—although awareness in itself is a change. What part expands during the inhale: your shoulders, chest, diaphragm (at the bottom of your ribs), stomach? Is there a pause or rush of air as you exhale? How much air is still in your lungs as you breathe in again?

Just breathe, in . . . out . . . for five breaths. Continue with this as long as you'd like, coming back to awareness of your body breathing if your mind wanders away.

Pause

You might find a tiny little no-breath pause at the end of your exhale and/or at the end of your inhale. It can be a lovely moment in the breath cycle, a few seconds of empty stillness before movement continues. Take a cycle of four or more breaths just to notice these no-breath pauses.

Length of Breath

Count your breath: the inhale (one-two-three-four . . . however long it is), then the exhale. You may find that the inhale and exhale are the same, or that one is longer. It's been said by yogis that in order to relax, one should take a longer exhale than inhale.

Here's how: using a medium-slow pace, count to four, five, or six on your inhale, then to eight, nine, or ten on your exhale. Some suggest a one-to-two ratio—for instance, three counts on inhale and six counts on exhale.

Play with the rhythm so it suits your body on this night. (Each night has its own rhythm.)

If you'd like, add a few counts between the inhales and exhales for the pauses. A breath cycle might look like this:

Inhale *(one . . . two . . . three . . . four . . .)*
　　Pause *(one . . . two . . .)*
　　　　Exhale *(one . . . two . . . three . . . four . . . five . . .*
　　　　six . . . seven . . . eight)
　　　　　　Pause *(one . . . two . . .)*
Inhale *(one . . . two . . . three . . . four . . .)*
. . . and so on.

Breathing and turning the head: This helps focus on the breath and the gentle movement of releasing the neck. Lie in bed on your back, with your face toward the ceiling. Inhale as you slowly turn your head to the right—don't strain your neck. Once there, exhale. Inhale as you slowly turn your head back to center, and then exhale. Do the same to the left. Repeat the cycle two to five times. Then just breathe.

Alternate-Nostril Breathing

Many yogis consider alternate-nostril breathing to be one of the best techniques to calm the mind and the nervous system. Some scientific studies have found that we have a natural cycle of alternate-nostril breathing that may boost our brain hemispheres and our thinking.

To do alternate-nostril breathing, breathe in through one nostril, exhale through the other nostril, and then reverse. Here's how: Sit or lie comfortably. Take the index and middle fingers of the right hand and fold them down. (You can use either hand, but I'm using the right hand for simplicity.) Exhale the air from your lungs. Close your right nostril with your thumb, and breathe in smoothly to a count of four through eight through your left nostril. Close your left nostril with your ring finger, simultaneously release your thumb, and exhale through your right nostril for the same count. Then reverse the process, inhaling through your right nostril and exhaling through the left.

Do three or more complete cycles using whatever count allows for comfortable, smooth breaths. (Sometimes you can do this with a stuffy nose or cold, but don't force it.) You can include a pause before you inhale and/or exhale if you'd like. After you have completed your cycles of breathing, drop your hand and take three breaths with both nostrils. Several people have told me alternate-nostril breathing clears the round-and-round thoughts in the brain.

Twists

Twists release muscle tension, realign the organs, and help with digestion, according to yogis. Usually, I think of my organs only if they're gurgling, so it's nice to connect with them in health.

These twists need no exertion. You don't have to involve your neck (especially if it's tender). You're simply letting your hips and shoulders unwind in opposite directions, then reversing the motion. Skip this pose if you have problems with your back or hips.

Lie on your back, and place your left foot on the bed near your right knee so the left leg is bent and the right leg is straight. Keep your left knee raised. Shift your hips a few inches to the left, and then let your left knee roll across your body, while your left foot stays on or near the bed. Your left knee may or may not touch the bed, and you can prop it up with a pillow if that's more comfortable. If you'd like, put your right hand on your left knee to give a little more pull. Stretch your left arm to the side. If your neck feels healthy, lift your head an inch or two off the bed, turn it gently to the left, and then lay it back down on the bed. Let your left shoulder relax toward the earth.

Take four aware breaths to let the twist gently unwind your body. Then roll your head back to center. Lengthen your spine on an inhale. As you exhale, realign your legs back to center. Shift your hips back to the middle. Take a few aware breaths. Then do the twist on the opposite side, bending your right leg and shifting the other way.

If you want to do a more subtle twist while sharing a bed, you don't need to shift your hips (or shift them as far), nor do you need to stretch out your arm (across your partner's face?!). You can even just cross your ankles instead of bringing your knee up. If you're concerned about stealing covers, put a separate blanket on yourself before you twist.

Hip Openers

After sitting all day, our hips hold a lot of tension. While yoga hip openers can be strenuous, the Night Yoga versions are gentle. Use your body as your guide. Back out of the stretch if anything hurts. If you have instability in the hip joint or sacrum, check with a yoga teacher or another instructor about strengthening exercises before doing hip openers.

Again, use pillows or blankets for support as needed. In fact, you might want to *over*-support yourself and feel held. Use a separate blanket if you're sharing a bed (or a separate space if your partner's a light sleeper) so you don't have to focus on anyone but yourself.

Pelvic tucks loosen hip tension. Lie on your back with your feet on the bed, knees up. Inhale as you tuck your pelvis forward (that is, your public bone at the front curls forward and up to your heart). Release to a neutral position as you exhale. Do this several times.

If you have a healthy back, tilt your pelvis the other way when you release (making a small curl in the back). You just need small, gentle movements, and to stay in touch with your body. At the end of the series of tucks, tuck your tailbone forward before your final release. If you feel tension in your back, bring your knees to your chest and pull them gently toward you, to release the muscles.

Hip opener: Start by lying on your back, arms at your sides, legs flat on the bed. Slide your left ankle up the front of your leg to your right thigh, just above your knee (or if you don't have much room, slide your ankle to the front of your calf). Let your left knee extend out to the left to open the hips, while your outer ankle bone rests on your thigh. If you want a little more oomph, place your left hand on your left knee and push out. (Did I say gently?) Gently. For more opening, raise your right knee up, skootching the right foot on the bed toward your bottom. You'll have a triangle of your left thigh and calf opening to the left on your right thigh, supported by your right calf and foot. You can put your hands around your right thigh or calf, and gently pull forward as your left leg releases a little more. Tilting your pelvis will change where you feel the stretch.

Breathe with the gentle stretch, letting your muscles release at a comfortable pace. Take four to six breaths, and then gently let go and return to lying on your back. Become aware of how your body feels. Then do the pose on the opposite side.

Shoulder and Chest Openers

Do you know the feeling of an overpumped bike tire? That's how my shoulder muscles feel after a day spent working on the computer. Opening out—reversing that inward curl—engages underused muscles, relaxes overused ones, and opens up the heart to the moment.

To release the shoulders and chest, be (you guessed it) gentle. You're reminding your body to let go, not forcing it.

Shoulder shrugs. Lie on your back, inhale, and raise your shoulders to your ears. Pull them back, as if you're trying to acquaint the shoulder blades (gently, gently, gently). Count to three, or four, or eight; then exhale and lower your shoulders as you keep the blades moving toward each other. Then release. How does that feel? Does your body want to do it again? Go ahead.

Heart opener 1. Lying on a bolster pillow or rolled-up towel is a great way to unwind your heart. To roll a towel, fold a bath or beach towel in half across the short end, and then roll it up. Place it vertically under your spine, one end at your neck. If you'd like, try this pose without a pillow, or put a rolled-up towel under your neck. Let your arms release at your sides, and breathe. Feel the opening in your chest, ribs, throat, and shoulders.

Heart opener 2. Place the towel or bolster pillow horizontally, right behind your heart or where the back of a bra would be (imagine it, gentlemen). Be careful of your neck. If there's any slight discomfort, make the towel roll less thick, or put another rolled towel under your neck.

In either pose, breathe. *B-r-e-a-t-h-e.* Take four to eight breaths, or breathe for five minutes or longer—just to be in your body as it softly opens to the night.

Resting inversions. An interesting yoga principle is putting your heart above your head. This reversal is good for the flow of the body, and good for life. How would your life be different if you put your heart first?

Inversions at night are said to help you relax and change the to-do flow. Inversions are also helpful for those of us with jumpy or restless legs, or for those who sit all day. To do an inversion called *Viparita Karani,* rest your torso on the floor or bed while your legs are raised on the wall or a chair.

If you want to rest your legs along a wall, first make a comfortable spot to lie down. Get a blanket to place over your body, and if you're on a bare floor, lay a blanket out to lie on. If you'd like, put a pillow, a yoga cushion (a rectangular flat pillow about four inches tall), a cushion from the back of a sofa, or folded blankets near the wall, about four to six inches away from it.

Get into the pose by rolling into it. It's not as tricky as it sounds. Lie on your side with your back toward where you will lift your legs, knees bent beside you. Your bottom will almost touch the wall. Roll onto your back, straightening your top leg and then the bottom one, to be supported by the wall. Use those few inches between the cushion and wall as a little indent for your bottom. Adjust yourself and the cushion so you are comfortable, skootching away from the wall, or bending your knees if your hamstrings (at the backs of your thighs) or calves feel tight. Some people like to wrap a belt or yoga strap around their thighs or ankles to allow the legs to rest into each other.

Feel how delightful it is to reverse the flow of gravity. When Michael the baker tried it, he felt his legs breathe a sigh of relief and the tension flow out with his breath.

You can also rest your legs on a chair or couch. Roll into it from the floor, just like the pose with the legs up the wall. Bend your knees over the seat, or even extend your legs to the back of the chair. People who are experienced with yoga or shoulder stands can put their bottom on the seat, legs on the back of the chair, and extend the torso and head to the floor. However, check with your yoga instructor first, because you can pull a neck or back muscle if you're doing it incorrectly.

Now that you're upside down, notice whether your breath is the same or different. Perhaps it's smoother or has a catch. Breathe for a few minutes to absorb the experience of inversion, of breathing, and of letting go.

Restorative Yoga and Yoga Nidra. Restorative poses of yoga are useful to increase the relaxing parasympathetic nervous system, which reabsorbs those snappish adrenal hormones that can keep you tense or awake. Judith Lasater has taught and written great books on restorative poses, such as *Relax and Renew*. Restorative poses usually require arranging props so you can open your body without stress or stretch. Some of my clients keep a stash of props such as yoga bolsters, straps, blocks, and eye pillows, and do some of these poses when they can't rest.

The simplest restorative pose is *shavasana*. It is the last pose of a regular yoga class, also known as the corpse pose. Really, that's what you do—just lie there on your back, arms a little away from your sides. You absorb stillness and relaxation, and your body "saves" yoga learnings.

Being aware of relaxation is not something we usually do. Instead, we think we relax when the body is still, but the mind is nevertheless distracted by the television, computer solitaire, or books.

Learning to be aware *and* relaxed at the same time—that's the lesson in Yoga Nidra, a deep relaxation technique also called "yogic sleep." It's quite a change to relax the mind and just be. Classes may include visualizations or exercises. One Yoga Nidra exercise is to place one hand on the belly, the other on the heart, and focus on breath, touch (sensation of movement with breath), and light or images on the backs of the eyelids. You're not letting go into sleep; you're becoming aware of rest. It's a useful way to tone down the Conscious Mind to relax—and perhaps you'll sleep when you're done with the exercise.

Night Yoga

Michael knew that if he didn't do some simple Night Yoga before he went to bed, he'd be up and cranky much of the night. So he made gentle poses part of his Evening Ritual—some twists, inversions, and alternate-nostril breathing after he flossed his teeth and before he turned off the light.

Other clients keep a few props in their Night Nest and bring them out when the ache or tension in their shoulders keeps them from slipping into rest and sleep. Night Yoga is a bridge, allowing rest in the body without worrying about sleep.

Say hello to your body so you can say good night to it.

Chapter 8

A New Relationship
with Pain and Discomfort

I can hear my heart beating.
I can hear my stomach growling.
I can hear my teeth grinding and my joints creaking.
My body's so noisy, I can't sleep.
—Charles M. Schultz

PAUL USUALLY FELL ASLEEP RIGHT AWAY. Tonight he lay awake with ice on his shoulder, ibuprofen on his nightstand, and a frown on his face. He'd call the doctor if it wasn't so late.

Before bed, he fell in the living room and jammed his shoulder into the side of the sofa. His arm ached a lot when he moved it. Despite the ice, pills, and comfort from his wife, he couldn't escape the pain and worry: *Did I tear a ligament? How can I work tomorrow? It's getting worse.*

Paul hated any pain, especially on nights like this when it kept him from sleeping. He couldn't fall asleep on his back, and the ice on his shoulder fell off if he rolled onto his side. His wife dozed next to him—*She doesn't care.* The ice wasn't so cold anymore, but he was too tired to get fresh cubes from the freezer. His mind drifted to thoughts of the novel he was reading. He felt a little sleepy . . . *Will it hurt if I roll over?* He wiggled his shoulder to check. *Ow, ow, ow.*

Paul thought his pain was keeping him up, but his mind was waking him more.

Pain at Night

Bodies are wonderful. And irritating. Or both, at the same time. As I say when I'm sick, *Bodies: can't live with them, can't live without them.*

Irritations take center stage when you worry about getting a good night's rest. That tickle in your throat threatens to become a cough when you lie down. Your nose is still stuffed from last week's cold. You feel warm in the face. . . . Is your whole body getting hot?

It can be tricky to separate irritations from worries when you have medical problems:

- Rapid heartbeats, such as atrial fibrillation, may make you feel rattled and worried.
- With fibromyalgia, it's difficult to find an ache-free spot for rest.

- In early pregnancy, queasiness is everywhere—or the fear of experiencing queasiness if you roll over.

How do you sleep—or even rest?

During the day, you have TV, books, or phone calls to distract you. But it can be tricky to get away from pain and discomfort at night.

It's just you and your body. And your mind.

Pain and Discomfort

What are pain and discomfort, exactly? They're so familiar . . . yet hard to describe. It aches, pokes, contracts, spasms, stings, numbs, burns, itches, throbs, twinges, or tingles. What some call discomfort others call pain.

Hospitals use a number system to characterize pain: ten is excruciating; one is barely there. That's an internal comparison, since your spasm may be different from the spasm of your best buddy. (For ease of writing, *pain* in this chapter refers to a range of discomfort that Restful Insomnia clients have managed. These techniques do not substitute for medical care.)

Here are some things we know about pain:

- **Pain is useful.** It lets you recognize potentially harmful stimulus. Pain signals your body to protect itself from greater hurt and sends healing energy and fluids to the injured areas.

- **Pain is communication.** Pain creates signals so body parts talk to each other—and to you. For some, it's a wake-up call to connect with the physical.
- **Pain is subjective.** Paper cuts might drive you crazy, while your friend could dice her hand with paper and not care. But with headaches, she's a goner.
- **Pain is affected by your mind.** If you're worried and tense, you focus more on pain and you increase your reaction to it. In fact, the International Society for the Study of Pain defines pain as both the physical response (nociception) and the subjective and emotional reaction to it.

While all pain is not in your mind (hit your thumb with a hammer—it's not just mental), how you react affects your pain and even pain medication.

Research showed that pain pills were less effective in Alzheimer's patients because they didn't expect the medication to work. On the other hand, reduced pain using medication helps surgery patients recover faster.

What else helps manage pain? Visualizing and soothing your body, getting support from the outside (medical practitioners), and supporting your own ability to heal.

Discomfort and Suffering

Pain and suffering ran Paul's life at night, since he believed he couldn't sleep unless his pain was gone. His focus on his pain thermometer (*How much is it hurting NOW?*) kept him from rest.

While you might be less dramatic, it's a human response to want to control pain and make it go away. That's why you don't touch a burning stove twice.

When you can't control pain, what can you do? Change your relationship to it. As the Buddhists say, you feel pain and create suffering (such as anxiety, worry, and blame) on top of the pain. To change suffering when the body aches, reduce the stories about pain, change your expectations of pain, and relax—even just part of the body—despite the hurt.

Steven Levine, colleague of Elizabeth Kübler-Ross and the author of many moving books, talks about reactions to pain in *A Gradual Awakening*. The first common response to pain, he says, is resistance—*I don't want to feel this*. This may mean ignoring pain and doctors, self-medicating or overmedicating, or wanting something (a fourth medical opinion?) to fix it already. Resistance creates tension and stress.

What's the opposite of resistance? Surrender or acceptance. Does surrender mean pain "wins"? Actually, acceptance increases relaxation and healing, lowers your blood pressure, and relieves tension—all of which are linked to reducing pain.

When you let go of resistance, you soften both your mind and the area surrounding the pain. The pain isn't bigger than you; instead, your body and focus are larger than the pain.

It takes practice to let go of resistance to pain. Especially if the pain has been around for a while, scares you, or limits what you do. As you accept and investigate how you feel pain, you'll discover that:

- Pain isn't what you think it is.
- You can reduce the impact of pain.
- You can learn from the pain.

Pain isn't what you think it is. Pain often becomes a solid thing, like a shoe or a knife, especially when you're hurting. In reality, pain is a verb, an experience that changes. You can dance with pain, move around it, or move with it when it's not a *thing*.

You can reduce the impact of pain. As you watch pain, you may discover actions or thoughts that diminish the intensity of pain. For instance, if you have a moderately stuffed head, you can patiently breathe through the nose until one nostril becomes unstuffed, as the body responds to its desire for oxygen. A random itch—feeling urgent at first—may fade without scratching it, especially if you focus on your spinal cord. Turns out, spinal nerves, not skin nerves, trigger the itch.

You can learn from the pain. Ask if your pain has something to teach you. Are your muscles achy and immobile? The discomfort may be telling you that you need a rest—you're doing too much. If you lie down because it's what your body needs, instead of because the pain is forcing you to do it, you develop a more caring attitude toward the pain.

Soothing Pain and Discomfort
with Restful Insomnia Techniques

Restful Insomnia teaches you how to use your body-mind connection to reduce the impact of pain on your nightly rest. The techniques use the five steps of Restful Insomnia—the environment, body, mind, emotions, and natural connection—to teach your mind and body how to:

- Relax your body.
- Calm your fears.
- Distract your thoughts.
- Learn from the pain.
- Focus on your Spiritual Center.

Restful Insomnia doesn't suggest you turn into the stereotype yogi sleeping on a bed of nails. However, each moment when you're aware that you're more than your pain, part of you can rest and let go for the night. Managing pain and discomfort is a life-changing process. Try these techniques on the nights that you're bugged by your body, to befriend it again.

Relax Your Body

When your body hurts, you may feel you have no "home" inside your skin. Here are some ways to find a home:

- Relax your body from the top of your head down to your toes. Imagine a soothing color, the sensation of your gentle breath, a vibration, or a musical tone that comes from a healing force beyond your body. It moves into the top of your head and flows all the way down to your fingers and toes. It relaxes the comfortable areas and surrounds or lessens the intensity of painful areas. It creates a grounding cord from the base of your spine to the center of the earth, to send the pain to be recycled to healing.
- Notice areas outside of the pain. Do they have a different color, sensation, or tone? Spread that relaxing energy into as much of your body as possible, letting your painful areas be held by healing.
- Imagine little people or elves healing your body. They spray-clean your clogged sinuses, reknit your stretched muscles, encase your stressed joints in fairy dust, and put ice packs on your forehead. Again, a grounding cord can be useful to release what you no longer need.
- Ex . . . h-a-l-e. Then take two or three aware breaths. On the inhale, send oxygen around or into the painful areas, and release tension on the exhale.
- Try some Energy Medicine techniques to change the flow of your body's energy. Tap on your thymus (a few inches above your heart, where the breastbone protrudes). Or reconnect your hemispheres by alternating touching your right hand as you slightly lift your left knee, then your left hand to your right knee.

- Love each muscle and organ of your body.
- Try some Night Yoga, from alternate-nostril breathing and hip openers to gentle twists.

Soothe Your Environment

Ask for help, or use your Evening Ritual to be your own best nurse. Arrange your bed and Night Nest for healing. That may mean using extra pillows to support achy parts; clean sheets a hot-water bottle; available medicine and cough drops; and fresh water to support the healing power of rest.

- Clean out the room. During the day or night, open windows and clear out the day's discomfort or germs. Burn some healing sage, or spray some rose water (available at natural food or massage therapy supply stores).
- Try aromatherapy. Use an aromatherapy burner, or put some oil in lotion to spread on your skin. Lavender and chamomile are known to be helpful for rest, while mint has a stimulating quality. Even a little eucalyptus oil (Vicks VapoRub?) can open stuffy noses.
- Support or stretch your body with cushions: Rest your legs on pillows to ease achy or swollen legs. Open the chest by lying on a pillow that goes along the spine or at a right angle by the heart. Cuddle up to a favorite old stuffed animal for comfort.
- Play gentle, quiet music or white noise to surround you with soothing sound.

Calm Your Emotions

When you're healthy, it's easy to take the body for granted. But after days in bed with the flu, just walking into the kitchen can feel like you're trying for a gold medal in the Olympics.

What's your relationship to your body when you're sick? If you're stuck in anger or fear, it creates tension and distance from healing. Here are some ways to be more alive with your body, even when it's not behaving itself.

- Notice your feelings about your body being sick. Some people may have a long list; others may keep their emotions at a distance or hide them under anger, fear, or intellectual understanding of the illness. While it might seem silly, it can be useful to check out this poster of emotional faces (*www. easternhealth.org.au/champs/images/faces.gif.com*). See which ones resonate or look familiar to you. How do you experience those feelings in your body?
- Reduce the charge on your feelings by expressing the emotions and touching acupressure points. Escalate the feelings until the intensity fades. See chapter 11, "Emotions and Touch," to learn more about the Emotional Freedom Technique and the Tapas Acupressure Technique.
- Balance your anger by appreciating the parts of your body that work well. (It's easy to take them for granted.)

Restful Insomnia

- Talk back to yourself about your fears—don't fight them, but remind yourself that you don't know what will happen, that you're telling yourself stories.
- Focus on what you do know—the immediate body sensation of breath, skin, sounds, being present in your body.
- Write down what you're grateful about in your body and your life and why.

Diminish the Power of Your Thinking Mind

Paul's mind went ape over pain, and he needed to reduce the frequency or impact of worried thoughts. (Dr. Edward Hallowell calls them ANTs—automatic negative thoughts.) Here are some tips for giving the mind something else to focus on while you breathe and relax:

- Distract your mind by doing a problem. Figure out how many models of cars have ever been made; remember the names of all the yellow flowers; imagine each detail of driving from your house to the house of your childhood; count backward from 316 by sevens.
- Be an optimist. Imagine a positive future, and feel your whole body experience it as if it's happening in the moment.
- When an ANT arises, rewind it and imagine a happy time, perhaps from a vacation. Remember times of past illnesses that were healed.

- Use your mind to help your body get better. Visualize yourself swimming, exercising, or doing something that requires a little more effort than you're capable of at the moment.

Focus on Your Spiritual Center

Remember that you are more than what you feel, see, and touch. That helps you amplify the healing forces of nature, science, and the mysteries of life.

- Pray. Ask the forces of nature, God, or angels to open you to healing in whatever form it comes.
- Connect with your Spiritual Center as a healing guide or wise doctor. Ask what you can do in this present moment to increase your body's healing. Listen for the response—in words, sounds, feelings, colors.
- Read prayers—aloud if possible, even mouthing the words.
- Hold a symbol of healing or nature—a rosary, a sea-shell, mala beads, or a Star of David.

Be open to your Spiritual Center, and allow it inside in whatever form it is at this moment.

Paul's Journey

Paul appreciated the progress he made through his pain journey at night. He didn't become a stoic, but he felt a little more able to do something other than worry and complain about the pain.

Paul first created an "I'm Sick Night Nest" that included his pain medication, a heating pad, and some Bill Evans music. When he checked his pain thermometer, he stopped and remembered how his sore elbow last year got better in a week. If Paul's worries and stress took center stage, he listened to a healing CD.

Paul learned to rest and sleep in the night—knowing he could call the doctor in the morning, just to make sure he was OK.

And he was.

Chapter 9

Change Your Mind

Insomnia is a gross feeder.
It will nourish itself on any kind of thinking,
including thinking about not thinking.
—Clifton Fadiman

STEPHAN LOVED HIS MIND DURING THE DAY. He could keep up a clever conversation, got jokes right away, and had a virtual Google in his head. He'd earned his stripes as captain of a fisheries research ship in the Bering Sea—a difficult and dangerous job.

But he hated his mind at night. It would analyze work (*Do we need a new algorithm for measuring the migration?*), spew low-level anguish (*If my dog gets sick again while I'm at sea, should I fly home?*), or obsessively monitor his sleep time (*I almost crashed, but now I'll only get four hours*).

Thinking made his body jumpy, raised his blood pressure, and upped his tension. He liked the idea of sleeping pills to turn off his thoughts, but they made him groggy the next day when he needed to be sharp. If only his mind had a "standby" icon, like his laptop!

Stephan's mind kept him awake at night. He's not alone. It's easy to get caught in the spiral of thinking, carried away by stories that seem real and cloud perspectives.

The key is to change your mind, to detach the Conscious Mind's hold so the Unconscious Mind can step in to balance your body-mind. And how do you do that? These Restful Insomnia techniques help you reduce thoughts, increase awareness, uncoil repeated thoughts, untie knotty problems, and lessen blame. Additional chapters will help change your mind as well: chapter 10, "Resting with Meditation," chapter 11, "Emotions and Touch," and chapter 15, "Positive Focus."

It turns out there are lots of ways to change the mind once you recognize that you can.

Awareness Versus Thinking

What does your mind do when it's *not* thinking? Thoughts are pictures, movies, or ideas of life. Awareness is the real thing. Awareness is focusing on sensation. Thinking is *the meaning you give sensation,* commonly called a *story.*

I asked my friend Elizabeth to experiment with awareness and thinking by placing her awareness in the muscles of her derriere.

"I sense numbness and pressure," she said.

I asked what her thoughts were about it. "I've been sitting here way too long. I should get up."

She moved awareness to her eyes. "They feel heavy, like closing." And her thoughts? "Damn, I don't want to be tired. I have too much to do."

Thinking stirs up the Conscious Mind, putting it into high gear at night. Awareness changes focus so the Unconscious Mind takes over.

Take a little awareness tour of your body. Become aware of your little right toe . . . the indent under your nose . . . your left hip . . . your right armpit. . . . If you have difficulty making the transition to awareness, try placing your hand on the body part, and start with the sense of touching it. Once you have awareness, switch to thinking. Think about your toe, indent, hip, or armpit— it's a different sensation. When Stephan tried it, thinking gave him the sense of being outside his body. Awareness put him inside, in the blood vessels and muscles.

Stephan learned that when he withdrew his energy from the Conscious Mind and put it on the body, his mind slowed down. Some nights, he could simply place a hand on his stomach and remember, yes, he does have a body. Other nights, he used Night Yoga and Getting into Your Body. When he *still* couldn't connect to his body and Unconscious Mind, he knew he had to attend to the mind and untangle it. Here are some methods I taught him to do it.

Mind Eddies

Mind Eddies are thoughts and stories that spin and spin. They have lots of current and get nowhere—just like those little whirlpools caught between two mossy rocks at the edge of a river.

A Mind Eddy might be repeating an argument that's over and done. Or regurgitating what you coulda-woulda-shoulda done to avoid this discomfort you feel. Or anticipating an imagined argument the next time your sister-in-law phones about babysitting.

"What do I say to Jill? Maybe I'll tell her I have a date that night. No . . .

"Maybe I'll tell Jill she's using me. No . . .

"Maybe I'll say I have to work late for the next two months. No . . ."

And on it goes.

The Conscious Mind may think you're practicing a new way to respond. Which is occasionally true. But much of the time you're not even looking for any solution. You're on a little canoe in the river of thoughts, bouncing around against those rocks.

There are ways to get out of the river and rest at night.

Focus on Sensations

- Take the awareness journey around your body, mentioned in the section above.
- Focus on your skin, the air on your face, a little breeze running across your hands, the weave of the pillow-case on your cheek, the pressure of gravity holding you to the chair or bed.
- Return your focus to *one* sensation, as in meditation. It might be your breath (inhale and exhale, inhale and exhale). It might be the breeze running across your hands, or your heartbeat.
- Pay attention to the sensations that come from the Mind Eddy: your wrinkled brow, molars grinding, fists curled. Watch them ebb and flow.
- Listen to external sounds, from the train whistle miles away to your heater clunking.

Disrupt the Mental Flow

While it's generally not useful to argue with a Mind Eddy, you can still disrupt the mental flow:

- Sing. Singing disrupts the internal auditory channel, since the average person can handle only one sound track at a time. Try a song from childhood, an Ella Fitzgerald standard, a Christmas carol (even in July), or a commercial jingle. If you're concerned about disturbing your bed partner, whisper the song, moving your mouth to engage physical activity.

- Imagine you're in a theater, watching the movie you're rerunning in your Mind Eddy. *You're in the restaurant, repeating your phrases to Jill.* Now imagine that the theater quickly rewinds the movie—that you can see everything going backward and can hear all the dialogue and sounds in reverse. When the movie is back at the beginning, imagine putting an international "No" symbol (the red circle with a diagonal red line in the middle) across the image. Then imagine leaving the theater.
- Using all your senses, imagine a lovely, safe, relaxing place: remember playing cards with your grandmother, the green brocade of her couch, the edges of the deck as you shuffle, her voice asking about your day.

Movement and Your Spiritual Center

Put the Mind Eddy outside of your body. How? Take your hand and gently take the voice or image out of your body and hold it at bay. Put your other hand on your heart and breathe. You remember that you're more than this mental vortex.

Imagine your Spiritual Center. (See chapter 13, "Finding Your Spiritual Center," for more information.) Ask it to provide you an answer, maybe in your dreams, that helps resolve the spinning. Your Conscious Mind doesn't need to think about the mind eddy as your Unconscious Mind helps the wisdom arise.

Knotty Problems

Do you feel like you're carrying a Knotty Problem around your neck, especially at night? While Mind Eddies keep spinning without an end point, Knotty Problems need to be untied, sorted out, or clarified. You try to put the puzzle pieces in place: *I can't figure out how to pay bills and go to school.* Or *I want to be president of the PTA, but my wife is jealous of all the other moms there.*

Your Conscious Mind gets obsessed about finding an answer—that's part of its job description. But really, your Conscious Mind has spent hours trying to solve the puzzle. If it could come up with an answer, don't you think it would have done so by now? Your Unconscious Mind can help loosen your Knotty Problems at night:

- **Body wisdom.** Your Knotty Problem doesn't live just in your Conscious Mind; it also lives in your body. Take a tour of what body part reacts when you're thinking about the knot—your stomach, fingers, jaw, knees? Be present to the sensations, opening to them like a flower that slowly blooms.
- **Emotional charge.** If you have an emotional charge on this problem (and you probably do, which makes it tricky to solve), your brain keeps taking the same neural pathway to solve the problem. Think of it like a foot-deep ski track—not easy to turn out of. To lessen the charge and make the ski track more shallow, first notice the emotions in your body. Go beyond the

name—sadness, resentment, helplessness—to experience the sensations in your body that hold the feelings, as you might have done in the previous section. Then touch acupressure points as you intensify the sensations. You can learn how to do this in chapter 11, "Emotions and Touch," which describes the Emotional Freedom Technique, the Tapas Acupressure Technique, and other Energy Medicine methods. If you don't want to turn the page right now (I've had nights like that), put one hand on the back of your neck where it meets the head and the other hand on your forehead. This Frontal-Occipital (FO) holding helps soothe the body. Now intensify the physical sensations of the emotions . . . until they fade. Do it for just a few minutes to see if it works for you. (This technique helps many people open to new possibilities, but if the intensity is too much for your system right now, stop and write about your experience.)

- **Intuition.** Maybe you have the wisdom to solve the problem right now in your intuition instead of your Conscious Mind. You can access your intuition through your dreams (if you could only sleep!) and Wisdom Writing (see chapter 12). Or take a deep exhale, a slow inhale, and ask yourself, "If I already knew the answer intuitively, what would it be?" Drop into your body, and let your intuition appear, rise up, or speak to you.

- **Surrender.** Some Knotty Problems get tied up in the hope to have more control—over other people, acts of nature, or the economy. Surrender doesn't mean giving in; it means enjoying the flow of life as you play between what you can and can't control. The Serenity Prayer is a useful reminder to repeat as you consider your problem. (Substitute your own word if "God" doesn't resonate.)

God, grant me the serenity
to accept the things I cannot change;
courage to change the things I can;
and wisdom to know the difference.

- **Drawing.** Try drawing, but not in the usual way. Grab a crayon, pen, or marker, with both hands together or switching hands back and forth. This gets the hemispheres of your brain and body to align. Draw the problem—could be images of people, energy, emotions, or obstacles. When you're done, put your hands on your forehead and back of the neck (as in FO holding above) for three minutes. Now draw the solution. You may want to add drawing paper and crayons to your Night Nest.
- **Movement—with finger puppets.** Did you know your cognitive (thinking) and movement cortices are entwined in your brain? That's why you remember where to go, and forget why you went. Use movement to loosen the problem. While you can dance the problem out tomorrow, tonight try some finger puppets that fit on your fingertips. Buy some little dogs, people, or maybe monsters at a toy store or bookstore, or borrow some from your kids or nephew. When you use the puppets, each part of the problem speaks (or

whispers) to the other. Even though you're making the puppets talk, you're also watching the problem from an external viewpoint and getting more clarity. Those puppets might even kiss and make up at the end!

Blame and Judgment

Is it all someone else's fault? Is it too late now because you married the wrong person or got laid off or got stuck in traffic? Blame and judgments combine Knotty Problems and Mind Eddies to keep the anger and resentment going round and round and round while you stay awake.

A good way to unlock blame and take responsibility for your own problem (sigh, do I *have* to?) comes from the work of Byron Katie. She developed a process of questioning and transforming thoughts so you can learn to move yourself forward. You're the only person who can change (darn it).

The process involves writing your blame, usually in the form of judgments about someone who bugs you. Write how you want him or her to change. Then ask yourself four questions about what you've written to understand how much is a story in your head that relates to you, not the other person. Byron Katie goes into detail in her books on the topic, though this summary of the four questions can get you started.

1. *Is the thought really true?* Can you see, hear, smell, touch, or experience the thought outside of your mind? On the one hand, you can see wisps of steam

to know the coffee is hot, and you can feel tears to know you are sad. However, the thought *He doesn't love me* is your guess about someone else's motivation. You might know he ignored you, but you don't know that it's about love.

2. *Is there a stress-free reason to keep the thought?* Does thinking *He doesn't love me* serve you in any way? Instead of protecting yourself or getting revenge, you're likely hurting yourself.

3. *How would you feel if you let the thought go?* You can find new possibilities and resources when you're not in the maze of the blame or judgment.

4. *Turn the thought around.* How is this thought about you? Is there a way you don't love yourself? That's something you can change.

Changing your perspective on blame can be rewarding— and it takes courage to look at yourself.

Wacky Thoughts

My client Victoria couldn't stand those illogical wacky thoughts that popped up as she approached sleep. You know: *A knitted mustard green planet Jupiter rotates around a plastic Rockefeller Center.* She woke herself up trying to stop them, figure them out, or make them logical. The Conscious Mind does not like to lose control when the Unconscious Mind shakes things up!

I gave Victoria a few ideas to help smooth falling into rest or sleep:

- Focus on sensations in the body (the Restful Insomnia standard).

- Multitask, just like the woman who simultaneously drinks iced coffee, talks on her mobile, and smokes a cigarette. That means to let your Conscious Mind do its shtick *in the background* while you focus on physical relaxation or even counting sheep. It's a step in the right direction to drift in and out of rest.

- Roll your eyes, lids closed, so you're looking toward your nostrils, heart, or navel. As I mention in chapter 10, "Resting with Meditation," I've discovered that the motion of eyes affects thoughts. When you look forward, behind closed lids, your eyes will still track the movement of your thoughts, providing additional support to the Conscious Mind. Let's say you imagine your husband leaves dishes on the table; your eyes will follow the action of your thoughts, increasing the intensity of the issue. When you roll your eyes down, the flow of thoughts changes. And helps you to rest and sleep.

Let me add that eyes roll *up* when you sleep. However, many clients find it easier to roll the eyes down to release the hold of the Conscious Mind. The body will naturally move the eyes up when you drowse. Try rolling your eyes both ways—up and down—to see how it affects your body and thoughts.

Stephan's Mind During
Restful Insomnia Nights

Stephan found space for rest when he realized his thoughts about work and his anxiety were just stories. They felt real, and they colored his life, but they were not the complete truth. That little bit of distance had a big effect. Instead of pumping anguish into fantasies of work, his dog's health, or even sleep, he could just let his thoughts be.

It was as if he were cooking dinner while the television was on. He paid attention during the weather report, but he ignored the rest to make sure the onions didn't burn. If his mind rattled as he went to bed, he focused elsewhere during Restful Insomnia.

Chapter 10

Resting with Meditation

Meditation is not a way of making your mind quiet. It is a way of entering into the quiet that is already there—buried under the 50,000 thoughts the average person thinks every day.
—Deepak Chopra

I MET GREG AT A PARTY, and he asked me, "So, what do you do?" When I mentioned Restful Insomnia, I could tell by the avid look in his eyes that he was an insomniac. (Those who sleep through the night smile politely when I mention the program, then change the subject.) Greg and I talked about ways to let go of the chattering of the Conscious Mind. Then he asked me a question I've heard often: "Isn't Restful Insomnia just like meditation?"

"Yes," I told him, "and no."

He gave me a curious look.

"Restful Insomnia and meditation have similarities," I said. "In meditation you watch thoughts come and go, creating distance from them, which creates a sense of peace." He nodded. "Restful Insomnia has many methods to quiet or calm the Conscious Mind, including meditation techniques. However, practicing meditation in Restful Insomnia has a different intention than many other forms of meditation."

"What's that?" Greg asked.

"It's the difference between watching the thoughts in the mind to increase awareness and watching the mind to help it rest," I replied.

This chapter talks about those differences and describes meditation techniques that can help when your Conscious Mind keeps you awake at night. Your mind may continue to jabber, but you can train your mind to shift its attention much as you shift your attention away from traffic noise outside the window.

Let's breathe in, breathe out, and dive in.

What Is Meditation?

You probably already know how to meditate, even if unconsciously. That is, you know how to engage "in an activity that keeps your attention pleasantly anchored in the present moment," as Joan Borysenko describes in her book *Minding the Body, Mending the Mind.*

Maybe you've noticed the ocean waves while walking on the beach, then started to think about what to cook for dinner, then let your thoughts about dinner go as you focused on the rumble of the waves. Maybe you've learned to sailboard and focused on balancing, leaving thoughts of car repairs or other problems behind. Or when you've made love, maybe you've dropped your thoughts about the grocery list, and focused instead on your pleasure from comingling breath and rhythm.

Conscious meditation helps you to relax your mind, concentrate, focus, gain compassion, improve memory, inspire creativity, reduce stress, and more. And, as I mentioned earlier, it helps create distance from random, disruptive thoughts of the Conscious Mind.

And yet the power of the Conscious Mind is what makes meditation seem difficult, if not impossible, for many of us. The Conscious Mind loves to be in charge. It teases, cajoles, whines, threatens, dreams, worries, plans, spaces out, and moans—anything to get you to *quit that stupid breathing and get something done!*

In traditional meditation, when I'm sitting in a chair and focusing on my breath and the sensations in my body, I often find rare moments of quiet while my mind pursues its own agenda. It wants to be somewhere else, make plans, space out, wish people were different, and wish I were different. The Buddhists call these mind games the

Five Hindrances or Obstacles:

- Desire (wanting more)
- Aversion (wanting less)
- Restlessness (insomniacs know that one)
- Doubt (distrust)
- Sloth and torpor (inertia)

In most meditation practices, the intention is to watch the Obstacles, as if you're sitting on a mountaintop, watching thoughts of thunderstorms, tornadoes, and tropical breezes in the distance below. You try not to follow the mind on its wanderings. Or, more realistically, when you notice that you've fallen off the mountaintop into the rainfall or windstorm or onto the sunny beach, you return to the mountaintop via your attention to your breath (even if reluctantly at first).

So, that means when you're meditating, you sit. Even if you want to move to the other room because it's sunnier, you sit. Hungry? You just notice the sensation in the mouth and tummy and sit. Sleepy? Gently open your eyes, sit up straighter, and sit. Next time, if you start out sleepy, you may want to try a moving meditation (such as walking, tai chi, qi gong, or a dynamic meditation from Osho Deuter).

On that imaginary meditation mountaintop, you can connect with a presence that's larger than the mind (sometimes called no mind, awareness, or consciousness). That makes sitting, noticing hunger, and being alert a little easier.

In Restful Insomnia meditation, you also create distance from the Conscious Mind rather than be kept awake by it as you lie in bed. Most of the Obstacles of the mind come and go while you just notice them and breathe:

- Desire (wanting to sleep, to get up, to see what time it is)
- Aversion (hating insomnia, hating my stupid jabbering mind, dreading exhaustion in the morning)
- Restlessness *(These pillows are so hot; I should pee now so my bladder won't wake me later)*
- Doubt *(This 'watching my breathing' is a waste. I'm still awake; shouldn't I check my e-mail?)*

However, there are "obstacles" that are welcomed in Restful Insomnia meditation: sloth and torpor, also known as languor and inertia. ("I'm feeling *sooo* relaxed, I could hang out on this mountaintop, or wherever, forever.") With this obstacle, you gently tumble down into the valley of drowsiness, deep rest, or sleep.

Sometimes the Conscious Mind tries to catch you before you fall into doze-land if you become *aware* that you're falling. Now you're thinking, *Look, I'm falling asleep! Am I asleep yet? How many hours will I get? That's not enough time. Think of all the things I have to do tomorrow!* Off goes the mental alarm of alertness. Don't be hard on yourself; it happens to most people.

What to do? Return again to noticing your breathing and watching your thoughts. During the second or third wave of sloth and torpor, you might ride into that restful doze. For some clients, it's a direct route to sleep. For others, meditation techniques move them in and out of drowsiness—not ideal, but still better than a night of wakefulness.

How to Meditate

In meditation, you return your focus to your breath or body sensations, again and again, each time you notice that your mind has wandered off. That's why meditation is called "practice." Even the Dalai Lama has to refocus when his monkey mind finds a vine to swing on.

Here's how to practice meditating during the day or evening. Choose a time when you can be undisturbed—twenty to thirty minutes is great, although even a five-minute stretch is good. Choose one thing to focus on. The breath is a good place to start because it's constant, in the body, and softly moving. Other choices (there are about a million) include a body sensation, a mantra (a repeated phrase), awareness of one foot and then the other while you're walking, and the sense of extending loving-kindness around you.

- **Sit** on a cushion or chair with a straight back.
- **Close your eyes** or let them gently focus on the wall or floor a few feet ahead.
- **Settle.** Begin to move your attention into your body.

- **Focus** on your breath, a mantra (repeated phrase), loving-kindness, or the sounds around you.
- **Notice your thoughts.** They could be emotions, excitement, plans, dreaminess, irritation. Thoughts will come and go.
- **Return to your intentional focus.** Feel the experience of the inhale or exhale, the mantra, the sounds far and near as you notice the thoughts come and go.
- **Keep doing this until it's time to end.** Before you get up, spend a moment thanking yourself for meditating and imagine your calm awareness spreading to someone or something that could use it.

During meditation, your mind and body may experience many different things—relaxation or relief; review of daily experiences; released emotions; feeling antsy, creative, or bored; a momentary sense of quiet and peace; getting drowsy or dreamy; or finding new awareness.

It's all fine. Just watch and notice, including the sensations in the body. If your emotions seem difficult to sit with, use some techniques in Energy Psychology. (See chapter 11 for how touch and acupressure can take the charge off of feelings.) If you get restless, explore moving or dynamic meditations. Some other tips that can help your meditation:

- **Be present in your body.** Keep your spine vertical, sitting on a chair or a cushion or kneeling on a meditation bench. Release the tension in your muscles from head to toes. Try to visualize light flowing through your body.

- **Have an inner smile.** Imagine a small smile on your face to instill a sense of calmness and compassion.

- **Roll your eyes down.** With your eyes closed, look down at your nose and then toward your heart or navel. This eye movement, which I discovered as part of the Restful Insomnia program, works amazingly well to change the attachment to thoughts in meditation.

- **Release.** Some people feel the "release" phenomena—twitches, gurgling stomach, quivery body, or mental images—at the beginning of meditation. These reservoirs of accumulated stress drain over time, say meditation teachers Joel and Michelle Levey, allowing you to feel clearer.

- **Balance relaxation and alertness.** If you feel sleepy during daily meditation, open your eyes and softly look down in front of you. You can also press the tongue to the roof of the mouth and straighten your spine. If you feel antsy, focus on a calmer part of your body. Notice the sensations of restlessness as they change. You may want to walk slowly during meditation, aware of each movement of your feet.

No matter what, be gentle with yourself. When your mind is doing triple flips on its mental trampoline, kindly remind yourself to refocus. Gently. *OK, there we go with another thought . . . in-breath, out-breath.* When you yell at your mind, you're feeding its sense of power. That's true during the day or when you're using Restful Insomnia meditation at night.

How to Meditate in Restful Insomnia

I met someone who said she *loves* to have insomnia because it's a chance to meditate in the middle of the night. I'd rather just stay horizontal, but if my mind is frenetic at night, I will sit up in bed and meditate for ten to fifteen minutes. That changes the flow of thoughts and can help me calm down to rest—or sleep. Several clients also meditate during frenetic insomnia.

However, sitting up may be too much effort some nights. A student, Louisa, noticed the contrast between her mind erupting with worries, plans, and orders during insomnia, while her body didn't want to move. I explained the Restful Insomnia meditation techniques that can be used while lying down:

- **Align your spine.** This reminds your body-mind that you're not just sleeping; you're focusing on a new, restful perspective. Start by lying flat on your back (if that's comfortable), arms at your side, perhaps a pillow under your knees. If lying on your back creates any strain, lie on your side, and use pillows between your knees and even under your ribs to keep your back straight. Once you have the knack with

Restful Insomnia meditation, you may need to make only minor body adjustments.

- **Notice your breath.** The oldest technique in the world provides stillness, movement, and connection to life. Notice the flow of breath in your nostrils, chest, and abdomen. Experience each breath—the fullness, the pauses between inhale and exhale, and the release of air. Even while noticing your breathing, it's helpful to give your mind a task. Try mentally repeating the phrase *Breathing in . . . breathing out . . .* for each inhale and exhale. Or count each breath cycle until you reach ten breaths, and then start over again. Some nights (and frenzied days), I've shortened it to counting three cycles.

- **Repeat a mantra (phrase) or a prayer in your head.** It could be as simple as "Thy will be done," "Shalom," or "Peace." If prayers resonate for you, consider a Sufi Zikr, the Shema, the Rosary, or "*Om mani padme hum.*" It can be helpful to align the words with your breath: for example, "Thy will" on the inhale, and "be done" on the exhale.

- **Practice loving-kindness or Metta meditation.** Repeat compassionate phrases in your mind, such as "May you be happy, may you be healthy, may you be safe, and may you live in peace." Start with yourself ("May I be happy"), and then expand to those you love, those you know, those you dislike, and all beings in the world. I also extend it to the planet earth itself.

- **Concentrate on an image in your mind.** Do you have something that reminds you of a bigger pattern in life? It might be a cross, the Star of David, an image of the Buddha, a seashell. Imagine seeing the image, perhaps touching it. Or imagine yourself in a peaceful location, hearing a choir, waves, or chanting all around.
- **Focus on the sensations of your body.** Focus on sounds, touch, or internal sensations called *proprioception*. With *sound,* your ears are a microphone taking a "sound picture" of the moment. Start with hearing the sounds farthest away—wind, cars, a cat's meow—and moving in to hear the sounds of your house settling, your spouse snoring, the clock ticking, your own breath. Become aware of the silence that holds all the noise. With *touch,* notice the sensations of pressure, roughness, coolness, softness— whatever touches your skin. Stay slow, focused, and relaxed with each sensation instead of racing around your body to discover the variety of feelings. With *proprioception,* feel your body from the inside. Experience being horizontal in bed, the placement of your shoulders, the evenness or difference between each side of your body, maybe tension in your chest from working all day on the computer. Again, don't race; pause, relax into each sensation, and notice how it changes as you pay attention to it.

Visualize. Focused and repetitive visualization about the same image each time creates a meditative concentration and distance from the mind. (In contrast, a healing or re-laxing visualization may move to different areas that hurt or are tense.) One visualization is to imagine a flow of energy through the body and through the seven chakras, or energy centers.

- Imagine that you are connected to the center of the earth from the base of your spine—a grounding cord, chain, or beam of light.
- Imagine earth energy moving into your body via the soles of your feet up through your legs and body. (You might want to put your feet on the bed with your knees bent so you can feel the bed beneath your feet.)
- Imagine "cosmic" (or "I'm-not-here-all-alone") en-ergy entering through the top of your head. It flows down either side of your spine to where your ground-ing cord starts at the base of the spine, mixes with earth energy, and flows back up through your body. You can imagine the mixture sending any tension or stress down through the grounding cord to be recy-cled by the earth.

How do you find which meditation is right for you? Choose one, and practice it for several nights (unless it drives you batty the first time you do it). Sticking with one trains your Conscious Mind to reduce its gazillion reasons not to meditate or reasons to meditate *differently*. After you get into a habit, your body and Conscious Mind will notice and appreciate the calm. Then it's easier to decide which technique will be best for your Restful Insomnia meditation.

Beyond the Mind?

When Louisa started meditating, she asked me a half-joking question: *If I'm watching my mind or my thoughts, well, who's doing the watching?*

She had begun to shift in her sense of identity. *Am I not actually my mind, after all? This desire for a good night's sleep has taken me on a journey I hadn't expected.* Some sense emptiness or a void at first as their mind loses its illusion of firmness. That's letting go of ego, which lives in the mind and with which most of us identify. Many who stay with meditation go beyond the void to experience a connection with something bigger than the mind, bigger than themselves. It's not so easy to express in words (since it's beyond the mind, where words begin), though I've had glimmers of it in meditation.

Chapter 13, "Finding Your Spiritual Center," explores your relationship with something bigger. This can support your Conscious Mind as it learns new ways to let go into relaxation, rest, and blessed sleep.

Chapter 11

Emotions and Touch

Everybody talks about emotions,
but nobody does anything about them.
—apologies to Mark Twain

ISABELLE WAS MAD, MAD, MAD—fuming because she couldn't sleep, and furious at her neighbors. They had thrown *another* late-night party that didn't quiet down until after midnight. She had told them to be quiet by a reasonable ten-thirty or eleven, but clearly they didn't care or tell their kids. And they didn't answer the phone. Sure, it was Saturday night, but Isabelle couldn't sleep in past 8 A.M., and she needed her weekend rest.

At each loud conversation on their porch, slamming car door, or raucous giggle, Isabelle would stare at the clock and count the number of minutes she had been deprived of sleep. On top of that, it had taken her an hour after the last party ended to feel secure enough to relax again. How bad would it be tonight?

Isabelle's emotions were keeping her up—the car doors and giggles were just the triggers. The only way Isabelle thought she could control her emotions was to control the triggers. Then the neighbors didn't answer their phone or tell their kids to be quiet—*Ka-bow!* Her stomach grumbled, horrible pain returned in her right shoulder, and she could hardly lie still. Nothing to do but watch stupid TV until the party was done.

Emotions keep a lot of people up. The mental and physical intensity of emotions banishes sleep and dreams. A lot of people think that controlling the triggers—a messy husband, a micromanaging boss, noisy neighbors—is the only way to get some relief.

There are other ways to release the charge of emotions, including various acupressure techniques and Energy Medicine. This Energy Psychology, as it's called, releases emotional pain in the body. These methods focus on you so you can move into relaxation during the night or day and not find yourself yelling at the neighbors.

This chapter overviews the various techniques so you can try them out and see how they work for you. I have one important caveat: stay aware, and take care of your emotional reactions. If you feel nervous about doing these techniques alone, take the book to someone you trust and try them there. If you feel too emotionally vulnerable while you're doing the technique, stop. Breathe, write, let the emotions settle, and/or call a friend or resource to check in.

Again, I have used these techniques (once I got over the weirdness of tapping on my forehead or torso) to release the intensity of anxiety, anger, sadness—and even to break habits. However, each human being is unique; make sure you consider your needs when you choose the methods that lead you to a restful night.

The Truth of Emotions

My dad, a loving but withdrawn man, had intense bursts of affection and anger. He once heard a joke that made him realize how his emotions had a life of their own:

> One night, a man found himself with a flat tire and a broken jack on a rural road. He made a long trek back to a farmhouse, rehearsing what he'd say to the farmer: *Excuse me, I have a flat tire and a broken jack. Do you have a jack I could borrow?*
>
> As he walked farther, he thought, *What if he doesn't have a jack? What if he doesn't like strangers? What if he has a jack and won't lend it to me?* He approached the house, strode to the door, and

knocked. When the farmer opened the door and said hello, the traveler said, "Take your jack and shove it!"

This "Jack story," as we call it, shows how anger and other emotions spark a life of their own that grows and grows.

Where do emotions come from? Emotions can come from hormones, illness, medication, or food, or from a sudden incident or a recurring incident (getting dissed by a perfect-figure blonde, just like in high school). With all their triggers, emotions are primarily reactions to stories—mental images and dialogues. Emotions lead to a physical response. For instance, if your heart hurts, it doesn't mean you're having a heart attack. It could be grief, empathy, or compassion.

Are emotions true? They are on one level. If you feel grief . . . you feel grief. Someone patting you on the shoulder and saying "There, there, honey, don't feel that" doesn't resolve the sadness.

However, the story that's generating the emotional response—well that's often questionable, and may not be true.

For example, Isabelle was furious, panicked, and anxious about her neighbor's noise. The story in her head went: "They don't care about me, after how nice I am to them. I can't believe they're so rude. I can't function unless I have at least nine hours of sleep on the weekend."

No question, the story felt totally true to her. Having emotions and tension—a physical reaction—made the story seem real. But was it? It turns out her neighbors like her *and* they think it's reasonable to have a party until 12:30 because they can sleep through a fire alarm. It also turns out that Isabelle has gotten along after weekends of less sleep by taking a nap during the day. Not ideal, but manageable.

This logical understanding could reduce emotional pressure. (See the section on blame in chapter 9, "Change Your Mind.") However, emotions have their own inner reasoning that, as I said, feels true. Releasing the emotional charge helps open the narrow view of emotions—that the emotions *and* story are true—making it easier to rest and sleep.

Energy Psychology

Various techniques of Energy Psychology were developed and refined in the late 1980s and early 1990s. The techniques are based on the belief that touch helps with emotional healing, just as acupressure and acupuncture help with physical healing. These techniques work for many, and they're not harmful. Even though most of these techniques have not received scientific validation because it's difficult to measure changes in perceived energy, the techniques attract a wide variety of psychologists and therapists to help patients with their emotions.

Many people live *around* their emotions, skirting experiencing them physically. These techniques help you express and explore them, which usually feels good to the body (for instance, crying releases chemicals that peeling onions doesn't). Using these techniques alone or with a therapist broadens the narrow belief that since the emotion is true, the story is, too.

Here's an overview of how Energy Psychology works. (Details follow.) Focus on emotional sensations while you touch or tap specific points on your face, torso, and hands. The places are located on Chinese acupuncture meridians, but don't worry about getting the exact spots right as you start. For some techniques, you also repeat phrases while you touch or tap, to help change your thoughts and emotional reactions.

Before you start any technique, identify what you're feeling.

- What emotion?
- The sensation of the emotion. (In which places in your body does the emotional sensation reside? Describe the sensation as best as you can: tension, heat, coolness, numbness, color, shape, sound, or image?)
- Intensity of the emotion.

This helps you focus on the physical and emotional experience and helps you compare changes after you're done.

Tapas Acupressure Technique (TAT)

Acupuncturist Tapas Fleming, with her knowledge of traditional Chinese medicine, developed the Tapas Acupressure Technique (TAT) in the early 1990s to treat trauma. Tapas describes trauma as your system saying no or "I can't handle this" to a situation in life; "no" creates blockages that interfere with healing. TAT, one of my favorite techniques, is a simple and comforting way to hold yourself while you let sensations get stronger and abate. Here's how:

1. **TAT pose.** Lightly hold the following acupressure points:
   - With one hand, place the fingertips of your thumb and ring finger on the bridge of your nose, just one-eighth inch above the inner corners of your eyes. Place the tip of the middle finger of that same hand midway and about a half inch above your eyebrows. Those three fingertips are making a little triangle, with the bridge of your nose the bottom, and the top near the middle of the forehead.
   - Place the other palm on the back of your neck so your thumb is just below your hairline. When I do this at night, I just slip my hand between my head and the pillow, resting on that hand. You can switch hands at any time.
2. Focus. Focus your attention on your problem and the emotional sensations—wallow in them, intensify them. If you get spaced out, return to the sensation, an image of the problem, or the dialogue that gets your goat. If you're sad, repeat a phrase such as "I feel sad and I'm OK." That acknowledges both your emotions and the bigger perspective. Do this for five to

ten minutes—until it's hard to bring up the same intensity as you did early on.

3. Ending. When you are done, remove your hands, focus on your breath and body in the present moment, and take a sip of water. Go back to the emotional sensations you were having, and see if they still have the same intensity. Then ask yourself if you've learned any lessons from the TAT—anything from changing your perspective on people involved to realizations about underlying causes. Write those lessons down, if you can. Appreciate your courage to explore a new place in yourself.

For more information on TAT, check out *www.tatlife.com*.

EFT and TFT

Dr. Roger Callahan developed Thought Field Therapy (TFT), or the Callahan Technique, in the 1980s. In TFT, you touch a sequence of acupressure points related to emotional sensations of certain problems. For instance, to handle fear, you might touch meridians related to the stomach and adrenal glands. Gary Craig, a student of Callahan's, simplified the technique to develop the Emotional Freedom Technique (EFT).

In both of these methods, you tap—touch your fingertips like gently tapping a table—seven to ten times on points on your head, torso, and hands. Common points for both techniques include the inner tips of the eyebrows, sides of the eyes, cheekbones, middle of the chin, under the inner part of the collarbone, sides of the ribs about six inches beneath the armpits (where a woman's bra would be), the liver (four to six inches under the right nipple), and the insides of your thumb and fingertips (except your ring finger).

While you're tapping, focus on your emotional sensations and repeat a phrase such as, "Even though I have this [blank] feeling, I fully and deeply accept myself." That phrase blends focus on emotions and the bigger perspective, just as the phrase did in TAT. You mention that you *feel* rather than you *are* the feeling ("I'm feeling angry" versus "I am angry"). Remind yourself that despite your difficulty, you are a good person—even if that goodness is temporarily hidden from your view.

Do the EFT or TFT technique several times or until the intensity fades. Then you can rest, breathe, and take a sip of water. Write down the lessons you've learned.

While I don't delve into it in this book, the techniques also have additional movements that engage the voice and logic, and involve rolling the eyes. These are similar to the eye movement desensitization and reprocessing (EMDR) technique that has been used to treat post-traumatic stress disorder. If you want, here's a simple way to use the eyes to release emotional habits or stress: *slowly* roll your eyes in a large wide circle, first in one direction, then in the other.

For more information on Thought Field Therapy, see *www.thoughtfieldtherapy.co.uk;* for EFT, see *www.emofree.com.*

Resistance—Psychological Reversal

What do you do if the feelings don't abate—or if part of you is resisting change when you start? Perhaps you have a part that wants to stay in control, has the need to hide, or doesn't want to experience a related feeling, like sadness or anger.

This simple technique, where you rub spots on your upper chest and repeat a slightly different affirming phrase, works along with any of the techniques described in this chapter. It's also a useful method to do in and of itself.

To find the points, touch the indentations next to your shoulder joints. Move about one inch toward the center of your chest, then one inch down. You'll find spots that are a bit sore to rub. (Don't worry about finding the exact spots; the general location is also helpful.)

Rub those points in a circular motion while repeating a phrase similar to the one for TFT and EFT—for example, "Even though a part of me is afraid I'll never get over this problem [or my feelings of fear], I deeply and profoundly love, accept, and respect myself." Say this aloud a few times (or in your imagination while moving your lips if you need to be quiet), until your body feels ready to do a round of tapping or just feels a shift.

Donna Eden's Energy Medicine

Energy Medicine comes in many forms: Reiki, BodyTalk, craniosacral therapy, Matrix Energetics, applied kinesiology, therapeutic touch, Nambudripad's Allergy Elimination Techniques (NAET), and more. Since you can't see a practitioner at 3 A.M., here are some additional ways you can change your flow of emotional and calming energy during sleepless nights. These ideas come from the work of author Donna Eden, who is a joyous tour guide to the land of energy.

- **Tap your thymus.** If you are struggling to clarify what is your issue and what belongs to someone else (say you're worried about what your brother will think if you don't invite his in-laws to your party), tap on your thymus and create a boundary between you and what your brother will think. Tapping your thymus is said to boost your immune system. Your thymus gland is located above your heart, behind your sternum— where your top ribs join, a few inches below your collarbone. Tap on this area with your fingertips, using either hand, for about twenty seconds. To strengthen boundaries, raise your hand in front of your face every ten to twenty taps, as if you are creating a little "air fence" to separate your energy from others'.
- **Hold your forehead.** When you're feeling stress and strong emotions, this pose brings the blood flow back to your forebrain and away from your primitive and reactive brain. Lightly place your fingertips on the two bony protrusions on your forehead a few inches above your eyebrows; put your thumbs on your temples next to your eyes. Breathe. If you'd like, deepen

the emotional sensations for three to five minutes until they abate.

- **Smooth behind the ears.** Trace a line a half inch outside each ear on your scalp: start with a finger or two at your temples, and then slowly move around your ears to your neck. This technique is related to the reverse Triple Warmer flow—a calming movement that goes down your arms. If you want to do that flow, place the opposite hand on your temple, move it around your ear and across your shoulder, touch your elbow, and then move your hand down your arm out beyond your ring finger. You can do this two or three times—or more. It's also a soothing movement to do after Energy Psychology.

For more information about Energy Medicine, check out *www.innersource.net.*

Isabelle Returns to Herself

Isabelle was cynical about doing these techniques the first few nights after she learned them. She didn't want to stop herself from being angry; she wanted to stop the noise. However, the noise continued, and she thought she'd try Energy Psychology to see if it helped her be less touchy.

She started with EFT. Her phrase, which she thought a little stupid, was: "Even though I feel angry, I deeply and profoundly love, respect, and accept myself." It felt stupid to her because she *did* respect herself; it was her neighbors she was angry at. But as she repeated it, she felt more at ease. The tapping helped as well.

Then she tried TAT, and found that her anger turned into tears—a surprise and a relief for her body. She was sad, feeling lonely and unloved . . . maybe it wasn't all the neighbors' fault. She still wanted them to be quiet, but now she could do more than just focus on and react to the noise. She could rest into the bigger picture, feeling more at peace until the last partygoer went home.

Chapter 12

Wisdom Writing

Writing is both mask and unveiling.
—E. B. White

WENDY WROTE FOUR LENGTHY journals in the three months after she moved from Indianapolis to Seattle. She couldn't sleep with the bright streetlights shining through her apartment window, so she wrote instead: about her behind-the-scenes job at the public radio station, her unsympathetic sister (who just wanted to talk about her baby's poop), and her kinda-boyfriend, who had cooled off since he urged her to move across the country.

How could Jayson do that to me? He helped me rent a van—he even drove the van with me. He was so excited, and now he's just a stupid, cold, distant bore. He even canned our hike last week. I hate him.

She'd heard that if she wrote out her problems, they wouldn't keep her awake. But writing didn't make her feel more rested. In fact, she fell asleep only when she was too tired to hold a pen, sometimes with the light still on.

Lots of my clients were in her shoes—or in the middle of a journal—in the middle of the night.

Does venting tension on paper release the tension, as many insomnia experts say it does? Writing is wonderful—and getting a to-do list on paper can keep the Conscious Mind from chasing after details. However, when Wendy grabbed a pen and notebook during wakeful nights, she didn't seem to release anything. Writing the story of her unhappiness heightened the drama: *My boyfriend led me on. My boss doesn't listen to me. My sister is so narcissistic.* Solutions had a soap-opera quality as well: *I'll storm in and tell my boyfriend it's over. I'll sneak a longer lunch. I'm not going to babysit this weekend.* Tales of woe took root, building discomfort.

When I had chronic insomnia, I wanted to write. After all, I love to do it. However, I needed to find a new way to engage my Unconscious Mind, instead of feeding my Conscious Mind more active verbs, strong plots, and descriptive settings.

By focusing on my Unconscious Mind, body, and deeper knowledge, Wisdom Writing was born.

Wisdom Writing is a three-step process that taps into your insight. It's an easy, body-centered, and profound process in which you:

1. Reveal the core problem
2. Access your inner wisdom
3. Plan your next steps

Wisdom Writing allows the drama to fade to reveal the power I had in my life. But would this process work for others? In my classes, I found that it did. Students like Wendy told me they developed more clarity from ten minutes of Wisdom Writing than they'd found in weeks of insomnia journaling. Wisdom writing helps focus your attention away from the ramblings of the Conscious Mind and to the body, where the wisdom of the Unconscious Mind is revealed.

Here's how Wisdom Writing works:

- **Setup.** Snuggle into your Night Nest with paper, pen, and a gentle source of light (a glow pen, a dim or red lamp, a book light). Focus on your breath or one of your senses: Focus on skin, hearing, and breath, the taste in the mouth, or shapes and lights on the eyelids. You'll find an overview below, and you can get more details in chapter 6, "Getting into Your Body," and in chapter 10, "Resting with Meditation."

- **Breath.** Use the steady rhythm of your breath to become aware of your body, how your lungs expand and contract, the natural connection of life through inhaling and exhaling.
- **Skin.** Notice touch, first from the outside—air on your skin, pillowcase on your face, your knees pressing against each other. Then move to the kinesthetic sense of your interior—your tongue on your teeth, tension in your stomach. Focus on one sensation until your attention is ready to fully shift.
- **Hearing.** Listen to sounds, beginning with those far away, like traffic or an airplane. Then move to closer ones, like your dog's pant or the clock ticking. Then listen to the sound of your breath. Notice moments of silence; think of them as being underneath the sounds.

Steps for Wisdom Writing

I. Unveil the Core Problem

Let your body reveal the essential elements of the problem. Listening to your body sensations, images, and thoughts, write five to ten phrases or words to describe the dilemma. They could be names, feelings, body sensations, triggers, or associations.

For Wendy, the main issue was her boyfriend. Here's what she wrote:

Jayson

- Hurt and mad—my stomach is tight
- Doesn't he want me?
- Do I want to be here?
- I love him
- He said he loved me . . .

To be sure she captured the essence, Wendy returned to her body and breath between points and again at the end.

2. Tap into Your Inner Wisdom

Do you have a sense of your deeper or higher wisdom? Imagine that you already have a deeper wisdom—some people see it as a guide, sensation, angel, deity, or inner voice. If this connection is new (there's more in chapter 13, "Finding Your Spiritual Center"), imagine a gentle, safe, natural place. Use all of your senses: the image of the sea or trees, the sound of waves or birds, the touch of the sand or wind, the smell of saltwater or forest mulch, the taste of water or a berry. Invite your deeper wisdom into your body through your skin, the top of the head, or your feet. Feel the energy vibrate, see what the deeper wisdom looks like (golden light emanating out of you), and hear the sound or the silence of the deeper wisdom.

Let this deeper wisdom write three or more messages of support about your situation.

Here's what Wendy wrote after connecting with her Guardian Angel:

- Jayson really wanted me to come. . . . I wasn't imagining it.
- I'm glad I moved here, even if I end up moving back home if it doesn't work.
- Jayson had that weird shy time when we first got together in college.
- Maybe he's just freaked out about being in a close relationship.

While writing, Wendy focused on her body and breath between points and again at the end. She felt connected with what she was uncovering.

3. Unearth the Wisdom About the Problems and Your Next Steps

Imagine that your deeper wisdom or inner guide is a very loving parent who sees you clearly and tenderly. This is not your real parent (a human being with faults and foibles) but the Good Parent or Good Spirit that reminds you of how loving and how capable you are. This Good Parent notes your strengths, what you and others can learn from the dilemma, and perhaps what your next steps might be.

Here's what Wendy's deeper wisdom or Good Parent wrote:

- Wendy, you are creating a good adventure by moving here.
- You are learning a new perspective on life and your sister and family.

- You're taking care of yourself with Jayson, without wailing all over him like you did with your first boyfriend.
- You can talk to Jayson about how scared you both are about living in the same city again.
- You are a loveable, loving, creative woman.

Wendy was surprised at what she wrote: "Maybe Jayson's just scared instead of mad at me. Am I really loveable? Yes, I guess I am."

She returned to her body and breath with appreciation, some tears, and relief. She could let Jayson go for the night, knowing she could talk to him over the weekend and could handle whatever happened. She could be happy enough taking care of herself . . . a fact that made her relieved, and left her feeling a little closer to Jayson.

Transform your writing into a healing and soothing process.

Chapter 13

Finding Your Spiritual Center

The most beautiful and most profound experience is the
sensation of the mystical. To know that what is
impenetrable to us really exists, manifesting itself
as the highest wisdom and the most radiant beauty. . . .
This knowledge, this feeling is at the center of true religiousness.
—Albert Einstein, *The Merging of Spirit and Science*

DURING THE INTAKE PROCESS with my new client Jakelle,
I asked about her work, concerns, hobbies, dreams, and
spiritual life. "I'm an atheist," she said. "My mom took us
to church when we were growing up—even after my dad
had cancer. But I don't believe in God."

We talked about the several deaths in her family, and
I asked how she handled the grief. "You know, I have this

image about death," Jakelle said. "When we die, I think there's a part inside that rejoins the force of nature. Not like we're alone when we die."

"How does that line up with being an atheist?"

She paused. "Well, I guess I do believe in something . . . some force of life that's around us. Just not God stuff—too much killing and wars and people who think they have the only right view of God."

God can be a pretty loaded word. But your relationship with a Spiritual Center—be it called God, a larger-perspective, science, nature, Jesus, Mother Earth—allows you to rely on something beyond your Conscious Mind in trying to fix the world at night.

We talked about how to increase Jakelle's connection to her Spiritual Center to relax at night. "What do you trust?" I asked. She trusted that she would continue to breathe at night, see the sun in the morning, and most likely have coffee—probably a double espresso. "As you increase your experience of that larger perspective," I said, "you trust more in life, including your ability to learn and grow from difficult times."

Spirituality with Skin and Words

The war in Bosnia was a difficult time, and a little girl hearing bombs in the distance didn't want her mother to leave at bedtime. Her mom reminded her that even when she left, God was always with her. The girl replied, "That's fine, but I want God with skin on."

God with skin on? At times we all want to hear God announcing how the world works, clarifying what's your will and what's God's will. Sad to say, it doesn't quite happen that way. Spirituality is an experience, the ability to have a bigger perspective. It's not something that can be measured, wrapped in a ribbon, set on the mantel, or put easily into words.

But people do put their experience with God into words and into rules, objects, and meanings to create something they can touch—to remind them, they hope, to return to that connection. The problem is that the words and concepts, and not the experience, become the truth.

Given all that, I'm writing about God with the hope that you will translate my words about spirituality and a bigger perspective into language that applies to you and your nights.

Finding a Spiritual Center

Most of the time, I have faith in a larger, friendly, intelligent force of the universe. I wasn't always that way; my world used to be a scary place with a few nice things in it—some great things, actually, but I was sure those would be taken away. I protected my life more than I enjoyed it. I was cynical about spirituality, especially light-on-life people who transcended into "Universal Love" to avoid saying what they meant. (OK, I'm still cynical.) Death, injury, the state of the planet and the economy—life was a roller-coaster ride into hell.

And now? I still worry about the economy, the planet, kids, and health. However, those worries don't as often define how I see myself or the world, since I now have a different foundation. While there are no guarantees for safety, I know that the inner part of me—my soul—is cared for. My physical self is cared for, too, considering the situation of many others in this world. Having a Spiritual Center, I have *experienced* that I'm meant to be here, to be as useful and aware as I can be, and to learn about myself in the world. Your experience of your Spiritual Center may lead you on a different path. Nonetheless, it can provide a letting go and comfort so that you can rest your Conscious Mind at night.

The question remains: What does *experience* mean? Some say it's enlightenment, seeing God, or channeling an entity. Not for me. Through meditation, visualization, and exploring spirituality, I have:

- Remembered times when I naturally felt connected to the larger perspective, in nature or as a child;
- Imagined as if I could connect to Essence or Consciousness, which opened new doors; and
- Experienced my connection to the constellation of life.

Those connections, occasional as they were at first, expanded my reality. I could give my Conscious Mind a little break because something with a larger perspective was in charge.

For instance, when I looked for a job, my Conscious Mind said I had to be perfect (whatever that was at the moment). To ease the angst, I reconnected to a Spiritual Center, a bigger picture of who I am and how I fit in the world. I used meditation and a visualization to experience that peaceful picture surrounding me. Then I felt that Spiritual Center in my body, emanating a soothing vibration, and hearing reassurance that, yes, I am OK.

My Conscious Mind realized that I've been guided well when I trust the Spiritual Center, which helped me be more accepting of who I am, faults and all. It was much easier to find a job with that support in my corner rather than just my worried Conscious Mind.

When I spoke to Jakelle, I mentioned that people experience their Spiritual Center on many levels: as an idea; as an energy that flows everywhere in life; as being both inside and outside of oneself; or perhaps as an anthropomorphized form, like a Guardian Angel or Loving Parent. The view changes over time as you grow and as your Conscious Mind needs different levels of support.

Perhaps this is all new to you. Let's build and deepen the Spiritual Center that will help you rest at night.

Where Is Your Spiritual Center?

You'll find your Spiritual Center more in your body than in your mind. Sit or lie in a quiet place and relax your body, moving down from head to toe. Exhale and inhale at a comforting pace.

Remember a time when you felt connected with:

- Nature, a sunset, the interconnected patterns of growth
- A flow of life
- Deep intuition or creativity
- Other people or animals
- God, or whatever your name or image is of the larger forces

Remember the sensation you experienced then in your body. Did a part feel more open, more relaxed? How did your breathing feel? Perhaps you noticed a difference in the area outside your skin, or how you held yourself in space.

If you don't have a remembrance, that's fine. Pretend as if you did; how would your body feel if that memory were true—if it *is* true? Or imagine you are someone who does have that experience—a friend, a spiritual leader, or someone you create in your mind.

Bring that image into the present by imagining that you are guided and loved by a force in the universe right now. That force might be a sensation, sound, or color represented by the flow of nature, or an imaginary animal or person. To go further in your relationship with your Spiritual Center, especially when you have insomnia, continue with this visualization as follows.

- **Visualize a peaceful place to meet your Spiritual Center.** This can be wherever feels appropriate at this moment, though you can change it later. Imagine this place with all your senses, experience the details—the rough bark of a tree, flames in a fireplace, the smell of the cool air.

- **Imagine your Spiritual Center.** Ask your Spiritual Center to enter your space, through a door or from far down a path. Notice whatever details you can: size, movement, heat, sounds or words, even a name. Notice whether any areas of your body have changed with this connection—whether they're warmer, whether your heart is more open.

- **Talk to your Spiritual Center.** What would you like from your Spiritual Center? Reassurance, direction, an answer to a question? You can talk to your Spiritual Center and listen to the wisdom offered through words, images, feelings—even enveloping silence.

- **Ask for a gift or image.** Ask your Spiritual Center whether it might have a gift or image that would provide a reminder for you of this connection. Take it in your hands, if possible, and notice the details. When you're done with the visualization, you can draw the gift and keep the image in your Night Nest.

Then do a relaxation exercise (perhaps the one in the "Grounding" chapter, 14), and ask your Spiritual Center to give you a visualization of:

- A place where you can put your Conscious Mind to rest for a while, put it to bed, and keep it held in this larger perspective

- A companion who provides healing and relaxing and also reminds your Conscious Mind that it can let go
- A provider of wisdom to handle dilemmas that keep you awake
- A comforting force field to surround you when you are feeling stressed, or when you release with Energy Psychology

Maintaining a relationship with your Spiritual Center takes practice; without this practice, the Conscious Mind will start driving the van again. This is especially true when you're just starting to build the new spiritual connection. The Conscious Mind doesn't like change, and may dutifully inform you that connecting with your Spiritual Center is stupid, it's not working (you're still awake), or you're doing it all wrong.

You can set limits with your Conscious Mind without getting into an argument. For instance, tell the Conscious Mind that this visualization is what you're doing for tonight, or at least for the next twenty minutes. Tell the Conscious Mind that it can notice, but it cannot comment. Remind your Conscious Mind that you are a growing, capable person experimenting with your relationship with the Spiritual Center. The Conscious Mind will still be an important part of your life, just not the one always in charge.

The Conscious Mind will learn that it can gain from this relationship. "Spirituality gives you a purpose for living," says psychiatrist Todd Clements, "providing hope, calming anxiety and fear, and lending optimism to life."

It may take some practice to get out of your way and let the Spiritual Center flow, and you'll find lovely surprises from that wisdom when you do.

Forgetting and Remembering

Your relationship with the Spiritual Center will change over time; it will be crucial sometimes and forgotten at others. In the lifelong balance among all your levels of reality—from getting the kids to the dentist to spacing out to worrying about retirement—you may find even the memory of your Spiritual Center eclipsed. "Forgetfulness will arise like a smoke screen," says Ragini Michaels, a trainer in practical spirituality who developed the Facticity program. "It's just part of being human."

So how do you remember?

- **Habit.** Make meditation, prayer, or connection with your Spiritual Center part of your daily life or Evening Ritual. Most clients notice that it makes their days and nights a little easier.
- **Reminders.** People attach significance to physical objects to remind them of nonphysical spiritual experiences. Do you have a reminder? It could be the drawing of the object your Spiritual Center gave you, an altar on your nightstand, a rosary, or a picture of the ocean or of someone who guides you on your spiritual path.
- **Reading.** Wander through the spirituality section of a bookstore or library to see the range of writing on

meditation, prayer, visualization, even how the brain connects with God. Or ask your friends if they've done any reading on spirituality. You might be surprised at who says, "Yes, here's a great book."

- **Connecting with others.** Those friends or acquaintances who are exploring their Spiritual Center—it's helpful to have them around. Their questions and understanding help guide how your relationship with your Spiritual Center evolves. If you're the first on your block to look for a spiritual connection, you can find other spiritually focused people: join or create a meditation group; visit a church, synagogue, or mosque; volunteer there if you like it; or sing in the choir or in services—joining voices and breath with others makes the connections stronger.

Jakelle and Her Spiritual Center

After the Restful Insomnia class, Jakelle made a habit of connecting with her Spiritual Center every night, right after she turned off the light. At first, she felt a little silly, but after she hung out with her Spiritual Center for a few weeks, she felt more unreserved. It wasn't just "me against the world." She had a sense that she was going for a ride in life as well as steering. She could kick back, relax, and rest or sleep at night, held by something bigger than herself. It didn't matter whether she could prove that her images were "real"—they worked.

Chapter 14

Grounding

Putting your hands in the earth is very grounding,
if you'll excuse the pun.
—John Glover

WHERE ARE YOU?

Are you sitting in a chair, riding a bus, sprawled in bed? No matter where you are, an inescapable force surrounds you: gravity. Gravity helps you experience your body and connects you to the street, neighborhood, city, country, and planet.

You take the sensation of gravity for granted unless you're trying on stilettos, climbing out of the pool, or tripping over a toy. Nonetheless, connecting to gravity—

often called "getting grounded"—helps you remember that you're traveling on the earth and not scattered throughout the universe. During the day, you might get grounded by doing yoga, running, or noticing bumps in the road as you drive.

At night, grounding connects you to your natural self. It moves you toward the physical experience of sleep and rest, your Unconscious Mind, and the five steps of Restful Insomnia.

Experience Gravity

Suzie was a space cadet, always chasing the bright, shiny ideas shown in the ever-changing movies of her mind. Conversations were a myriad of tangents, from the architecture of the new building to the lint on a friend's sweater to the rice noodles in the soup she had for dinner. Lately, Suzie often forgot to go to bed, and when she remembered, her mind wouldn't turn off for hours.

Suzie learned how to ground herself by noticing gravity, creating a grounding cord for her body, and imagining the energy flow in her sleeping space through Intuitive Feng Shui.

You can experience grounding, too. Start by feeling the obvious pull of gravity on your body. Notice your butt against the bed or touching the chair. Is your elbow resting on the tabletop? Are your fingertips supporting the weight of your head? Is your shoulder curled under the pillow? Do you feel more pressure in one part of your body than another?

Each person's body manages gravity in subtle and unique ways. Try this: Sit straight on the chair, or lie on your back without a pillow. Take a few breaths to become aware of your whole body, resting in space. Now see if you can notice a difference between each side of your body, perhaps different pressure points (for example, your left ribs may press on the mattress, but just your right shoulder blade). Does one side feel heavier, more dense, or more spread out? If you were to get up, to which side would you roll? If you turn your head slightly to the right, how does the rest of your body react?

Play with how subtle shifts change your sense of your body as a whole. In fact, Moshé Feldenkrais discovered a whole system of somatic body movement when he was immobilized with knee problems, which led him to create the Feldenkrais work.

If certain positions feel more restful, they may be your most natural way to sleep or rest. Or you may discover unexpected body postures (even lying down) that help you relax.

Create a Grounding Cord

Suzie deepened her tie to the earth through the following exercise, which I provided in the Restful Insomnia class she attended.

See, hear, or imagine a line—a grounding cord—connecting your body to the center of the earth. The line might be a cord or rope, a beam of light, a sound wave, or a vibration.

The grounding cord starts in the center of the body near the bottom of your spine. The cord can be made from light, sound, or vibration; it travels down through your chair, bed, carpet, floor, building foundation, crust of the earth, and deep into the earth's center. Some clients find that their cord wiggles or can't go down to the center. In that case, I suggest they envision roots growing into the earth, like a giant oak tree's. They can connect to the center of the earth later, if they desire.

The grounding cord reminds you and your body of being safely connected to the planet. Meanwhile, the earth energy *enters* your body through your feet, completing the loop with the grounding cord. To feel this if you're sitting, place your feet on the floor; if you're lying down, raise your knees, and place your feet on the mattress. Feel your soles. Imagine the energy of the earth entering your feet. You may experience a color, vibration, tone, or scent working its way up through your legs.

Let the earth energy rise up through your feet, legs, and hips. Then notice as it flows back down through the grounding cord where it attached near the base of your spine. That circle of energy—coming up your legs and down through the grounding cord—helps you sense the earth supporting you, just as the earth supports an oak tree.

Clear Out Stuck Places

Clear out places in your body that are tense, numb, or stuck, to release into Restful Insomnia. Use the grounding energy you've already created, incorporated with universal or Spiritual Center energy.

I learned this technique from a trained psychic friend. It took some getting used to, but it combined my imagination with experience in my body. I like it, and so do many of my clients.

Imagine universal energy coming down through the top or crown of your head and then flowing down your body on either side of your spine. When it reaches the bottom of your spine, it mixes with the earth energy arising through your feet. Then the mixture flows up the front of your spine. Some of the mixture can flow out the top of your head and hands, while the rest flows back down and out the grounding cord.

This energy clears out tension in your body you're holding in your muscles. You can also imagine it clearing out your energy centers, also called *chakras*. Chakras are points in a body's energy system; the concept comes to us from India. You have seven main chakras aligned throughout your body, a few inches in front of your spine.

The first chakra is located where your grounding cord connects to the base of the spine. It is associated with survival and the color red.

The second chakra is located a few inches below your navel and a few inches in. It is associated with emotions and the color orange.

The third chakra is located in the solar plexus, between the lower parts of your lungs. It is associated with the sense of power and the color yellow.

The fourth chakra is located around the heart. It is associated with love, with integrating the body and spirit, and with the color green.

The fifth chakra is located just behind the indentation where your collarbones meet, in the lower throat. It is associated with communication with yourself and others and the color blue.

The sixth chakra is located within the middle of your forehead and is also called the "third eye." It is associated with knowing, vision, and the color purple.

The seventh chakra is located just at the top of your head where a baby's fontanel is and where the universal energy enters. It is associated with spiritual connection and the color violet.

You also have chakras, or energy points, in your palms and soles, among other places. Clearing these can help increase your connection to the earth, productivity, and creativity.

Recycle and Renew

Where does all this tension, stuckness, and unneeded energy go? It flows back down your body (via the channels on either side of the spine), through your grounding cord, and to the center of the earth. The earth recycles your unneeded or cleared energy, just as an old piece of aluminum can turn into something useful to someone else.

Any energy you need will come back to you through the grounding flow, renewed and revitalized.

Ground Your Space

Not only can you ground your body; you can ground your room or house, too. Visualize a grounding cord coming from the corners of the floor, meeting in the center of the room, and then going down into the earth. When Suzie tried this, it made her more aware of her environment. Then Suzie cleared the energy in her space through the grounding cord as well.

Imagine something pleasant—say, a golden rose—entering the room from a corner of the ceiling. The rose floats through the room and magnetically gathers up old unneeded or toxic energy that may still linger in your space—an argument, bad dream, illness, or scared child. When the rose has gathered its fill, it goes down the grounding cord for recycling. Use as many roses as it takes you to create a safer, clearer space.

Restful Insomnia Grounding

When Suzie grounded her body and room, she strengthened her connection to her natural self. She became closer to the rhythms of her body as the Conscious Mind took a break.

When you are grounded in your body at night, you are experiencing the natural connection to rest and renewal.

Chapter 15

Positive Focus

If you don't get everything you want,
think of the things you don't get that you don't want.
—Oscar Wilde

ROSE-COLORED GLASSES? Not on my client Jasmine. While she's nice, kind, and smart, she notices the flaws in life before she sees the good. After a dinner date with her husband, for example, she'll first mention what she didn't like (the soup was too salty, and the waiter forgot her wine), and then she'll talk about what she did (the halibut with hazelnuts was superb, and they'll definitely go back for their anniversary).

She doesn't think of herself as glum. She's a creative person who meets challenges by first seeing what's wrong in a situation. She persistently looks for problems to overcome, like salty soup and no wine. By checking the mantel of her life with a white glove, all she sees is dust—especially in the night, when her mind is a whirlwind of problems.

I know how she feels—I love solving problems, too. That's why I developed Restful Insomnia. But in trying to make the future better than the past, or to make the present meet my expectations, I often miss the happiness of being alive to what's going on right now.

I tried the positive-affirmations routine—it sounded great in theory. Sure, thoughts can influence the body, energy, and even what happens to me. However, my body, energy, and what happens also influence my beliefs and my thinking. Could my Conscious Mind actually run everything? Did I really want to be positive all the time? Is that even realistic?

Something else was required, something else that balanced the body and the mind.

To let go of my love affair with the negative (Godzilla stalking my insomnia mind), I played with Positive Focus on many levels, from virtues, writing, Paradox Management, and Energy Psychology to experiencing the positive in my body.

This Positive Focus integrates the mind, body, and spirit. It has made me and my clients more restful at night, more present during the day . . . and then more able to let go the next night.

Practice one or two of these tips for a few nights. If they resonate with you, include them in your Restful Insomnia program. They'll change your nights and days.

Inner Smile

By now, most people have heard that emotions influence the body and that the body influences emotions. Much came to light with the research of Paul Ekman, who studied emotions and faces. When he and a colleague created a photo collection of facial expressions (they moved each muscle of their faces individually, sometimes with a string in the skin—yuk!), they found that their expressions influenced their moods. After a day of angry grimaces, Dr. Ekman and his cohort felt grumpy for hours and had matching bodily responses—increased pulse rate, blood pressure, and body tension—just as if a car had cut them off on the freeway.

The interconnection between the body and emotions has gained insight from some reactions to Botox injections. I read about an anxious woman who didn't respond to medication for her fears. However, she did relax when Botox eliminated her ability to squeeze her brows together. The perpetual furrowing of her brow had fueled her anxiety.

It's not just scientists or Botox providers who know how the body influences the mind. Thich Nhat Hanh, a renowned Vietnamese Zen Buddhist teacher, encourages his students to create an inner smile during meditation and in daily life. It's a little smile that involves the lips, cheeks, and eyes.

That silly little inner smile instantly changed Jasmine's perspective. During class, we practiced looking at a stranger with our eyes narrowed in critical judgment: "That guy looks like a jerk." Then we made a gentle, barely noticeable inner smile, looked at the same guy, and said, "He looks like a jerk." But the phrase didn't have the same pull or oomph. It was more like, "Yeah, he might be a jerk, but so what?"

You don't need to look like a posing celebrity. Just practice a gentle inner smile in the eyes and mouth—or even a gentle nod of the head like a *yes*—and you'll find that your perspective changes, adding a layer of acceptance to the current reality and struggles of life.

Gratitude

When you've been laid off, it's easy to skip over appreciation for hot running water, health, friends, and family. Although gratitude won't get you rehired or make Jasmine's waitress serve faster, it does provide balance. Though you may still be mad at the results of rampant greed, you're at least happy you've paid off your car loan.

The habit of expressing gratitude brings you more moments of thankfulness and contentment, and can help you let go into rest—even sleep. Gratitude plants seeds from a perspective of contentment—a healthier compost for the flowering of your ability to meet life's challenges.

One of the best times to get into the habit of gratitude is during your Evening Ritual or before you turn off the light. Write three or more things that you feel grateful for that happened during the day, including why they made you happy. Over time, you'll become more aware of your unique values.

Jasmine's list includes the following:

- Sunshine! Color, space, expanse, and light.
- Going for a walk: feeling my body move, being outside.
- Having a clean house: organization, expanse in the rooms, containment of stuff.

Jasmine can see from her list that she values expanse, movement, and light. Which is good to know when she needs a boost during the day or when she's planning her next job or vacation.

Gratitude Is a Verb

Is gratitude just a thank-you note?

> *Dear Higher Power / Natural Wisdom / God,*
>
> *Thank you for the nice sunset, my car, my kids.*
>
> *Signed, Me*

While it is nice that you have things, that's not the purpose of life. It's also nice to remind yourself of the experience of being alive, being conscious, making choices, and turn gratitude into a verb.

- "I'm thanking you for being able to see the orange and purple sunset."
- "I'm grateful for experiencing the relaxation of driving a paid-off car."
- "I'm grateful for being a mom and learning how to love and learn from my kids."

Including actions moves your gratitude from *having* to *being*. You can be grateful for your movement through life—and your movement through the night.

I know that the word *grateful* comes from the root *gratitude,* but I think it should be spelled *greatful.* Don't you agree?

Inviting the Energy of Virtues

During difficult times, it's easy to misplace not only gratitude but also your own good qualities. The inner critic loudly defines how aloof, lazy, messy, or mean you are—right down to the words you said or the keys you lost. When this happens, your kindness, hard work, and warmth get lost.

Balance the worry and negativity of the night with experiencing the energy of virtues. What are virtues? *Prudence, justice, temperance,* and *fortitude*—those are the words Plato used (but in Greek). In common English, virtues range from *assertiveness, cleanliness, detachment,* and *humility* to *purposefulness*—following the list compiled by the Virtues Project. But those words are just concepts until you experience them in your body, as Jasmine did.

In addition to persistent negative thinking, Jasmine was a time-twit. If her husband wanted to check his e-mail when she was ready to leave the house, steam would erupt from her ears. And traffic? She gave herself *exactly* enough time to get to her destination and never had any leeway to mess with even the usual traffic jams, much less being behind a fender bender.

"Be a little patient," her husband would suggest.

Patient? That word had no meaning when she was in a rush, whether she was in traffic or trying to go to sleep as the numbers on the clock transformed from 1:28 to 2:43. What was the value of patience? Jasmine had no idea. I suggested she try a few of the following options:

- Imagine someone who is patient, and pretend to be him or her.
- Go to a clothing store and try on "patient" clothes (whatever they would look like).
- Experience how your body feels in a rush; locate one tiny area that feels more patient than the rest, and let that energy grow.

Jasmine couldn't imagine being a patient person, but she imagined her patient cat. Jasmine closed her eyes, relaxed, and pretended to be her cat . . . just lazing, waiting, sniffing, resting. It made her think of sitting in the sun at the beach all afternoon, of the end of a good meal with her husband, and of strolling through a bookstore. I asked her to describe what it felt like in her body. "Still on the outside, kind of blue gray, and waves on the inside, slow vibration," she replied. That description helped her identify the sensation.

She continued to describe how her body felt different when she was rushing: "It feels like the outside of my body is vibrating very quickly, with sharp edges, and the inside has almost disappeared." She understood, with a bit of sadness, how much she lost herself in the rush. She let her body absorb the energy of *patience* until she had a deep experience of the sensation.

Now, a few months after Jasmine started experiencing patience every few nights, she is not quite as compulsive in being a time-twit. She can feel the slower vibration of patience at a stoplight, and she allows herself to be a little late for nonurgent errands. At night she can now spend ten or fifteen minutes not watching the clock (a good beginning). Patience has expanded her awareness, so she has more options.

Moving Through the Paradox of Life

Can you always live in virtues? Maybe if you live in a cave and don't interact with the world. But out here, in real life, we live in a world of opposites—duality or paradox, as the mystics say. Understanding how to move through opposites helps you let go of struggles during insomnia.

It's easy to think of tangible opposites like big and small, night and day, up and down. But if you describe the process of life—"I'm married, with a teenager, and am in school to learn a new career"—you'll also be talking about opposites: married and single, parent and childless, changing and staying the same.

Any one of a pair of opposites requires its "other side" to define itself. Try defining *alone* without comparing it with *together.* Same for *trust* and *doubt,* for *success* and *failure,* or for *relaxed* and *stressed.* Heck, you couldn't breathe if you didn't have both an *inhale* and an *exhale.*

Making choices between opposites is critical for physical survival. You want to stay warm rather than cold, to be fed rather than starve, to be healthy rather than ill. It's also natural to apply that survival technique to mental and emotional life. You want to be *together* with someone, not *alone* . . . and *trusting, successful,* and *relaxed* to boot. Although it's a natural response to struggle to avoid *doubt, failure,* and *stress,* the struggle turns into what Buddhists call *suffering.*

They say we can't avoid pain in life, but we can reduce suffering. Suffering comes from our desire to avoid the experience of pain. On the one hand, if we anticipate pain and try to avoid it, we suffer: "I'll leave you first, so I won't feel bad if you get sick of me." On the other hand, we also suffer if we try to cling to a pleasant feeling: "Let's elope, even though we just met last week."

We all get caught up in wanting what we want, avoiding what we don't, and not trusting the flow of life. We even believe that if we don't get what we want, or if we get what we don't like, we must be bad. But let's get real: Stuff happens. There will be both pain and pleasure, and, believe it or not, that doesn't define who we are.

So how do we *not* suffer if we're laid off, alone, and doubtful? The knack is to learn how to simultaneously participate in and at the same time watch life's changes.

I've learned how to find some contentment as I've studied Paradox Management with its developer, Ragini Michaels. Not suffering as much means seeing how, no matter what I do, life always has clouds and silver linings. It means understanding that feelings come and go and that they don't define who I am—even when my lonely thoughts say, "I always feel sad and always will."

How does Paradox Management relate to Positive Focus? Instead of just focusing on the "good," it allows you to rest with what you consider "negative." Keep reading to see how to accept the positive and negative without losing yourself.

Paradox Flow

With opposites, as with the yin/yang symbol, the negative isn't all bad and the positive isn't all good. Each opposite has strengths and weaknesses. As we move through life, we travel from the strengths of one opposite to its own weaknesses; then we go to the strengths of the other side and then its weaknesses. Try this idea out, noticing how to move between *alone* and *together* in a relationship:

- You're with your partner and feel connected, companionable, and stimulated. Those are the strengths of being together.
- After a while, though, you start to feel touchy, spaced out, jumpy, and sensitive. Those are the weaknesses of being together and avoiding aloneness.
- You decide to spend some time alone. *Aaah,* sweet connection with yourself. You feel creative and in tune. Those are the strengths of being alone.
- Hang out in that too long, though, and you begin to feel lonely, rejected, and sad. Those are the weaknesses of being alone and avoiding togetherness.

The cycle continues as you move from being together to being alone.

Usually, you fight feeling touchy, jumpy, and lonely—feeling negative about feeling negative. An alternative is to understand the flow and relax, even when you're feeling spaced out, sensitive, or sad. Again, those experiences don't define who you are, though it's easy to think they do. They're actually just signals that it's time to make a change. *The flow of life wants you to grow and change, to renew, rebalance, and expand.* That's exactly what nature provides via the seasons—growth and expansion, balanced by decay and contraction. That may be one reason why being in nature makes you feel relaxed: nature doesn't fight the flow of life.

So how do you do this? The more aware you are—and your awareness is bolstered by meditation—the more you realize that while success, togetherness, and trust are ducky, those not-so-desired feelings of failure, aloneness, and doubt can also help you grow, be creative, and feel a part of the larger world.

Embrace, feel, and move through both the good times and the bad times to expand and appreciate all of life.

Re-dreaming Nightmares

Sometimes the negative comes at night, in dreams, when you're not quite up for embracing it. My recurring nightmare was that I was trying to land an airplane the size of an office building on a narrow city street while piloting from an outside balcony of the plane. I had this dream every few months, sometimes every few days, and each time I had it I awoke disoriented, adrenaline pumping, too scared to return to sleep. It didn't matter that I understood the symbolism of dreaming about feeling overloaded. The dream felt real, scary, and likely to happen again if I fell back asleep.

What changed my nightmare—that night and, eventually, forever—was re-dreaming the nightmare so that it had a healing, positive, restful conclusion. My friend Michael suggested that I try this:

Lie down in a restful position. Breathe . . . and envision the details of the nightmare. Now imagine a new and improved version of your inner experience, one where you:

- **Change the attributes.** Make yourself bigger or the scary thing smaller.
- **Become capable.** Find a rule book, get clothed, or make everyone else naked.
- **Get protected.** Bring in a superhero, best friend, or yourself as a wise adult to save you from harm.
- **Disempower evildoers.** Fire the teacher who's giving a surprise test, or spray a fire extinguisher into the mouth of the dragon.
- **Evaporate evil.** Sprinkle everything with fairy dust, which dissolves things or feelings you don't like.

After re-dreaming a few episodes of my flying-skyscraper nightmare (I made the plane smaller, hired a pilot, and envisioned magical dragons protecting the outside), the dreams got less scary—even fun once I imagined myself flying over tropical locations. Eventually, those dreams disappeared. And now I don't worry about nightmares, since I can rewrite their scripts.

Fears

Worry creates worry. Once your sympathetic nervous system is triggered, it turns on the stress response. Adrenaline and cortisol pump through your body, increasing your breathing, heart rate, and blood pressure. You may hold your breath, widen your eyes, feel hypersensitive.

Your sympathetic nervous system has a quick trigger for a fight-or-flight mode, keeping your senses heightened in preparation for additional perceived threats. At night, it's easy to confuse whether you're worried about something actual (an abusive partner), or whether it's the habit of fear (someone potentially breaking into your apartment, even though you're on the seventh floor of a secure building). A good book to help sort this out is *The Gift of Fear* by Gavin de Becker.

Toning down fear involves relaxing the body, de-escalating the emotions, and not just adding positive thoughts but changing your relationship to the fearful thoughts that may be running in your mind.

- **Notice your body and real life, right now.** How does the fabric of your sheets feel against your skin as you lie in bed? How does your body change if you exhale slowly for five seconds?
- **De-escalate.** Instead of trauma, turn the fear down to the level of inconvenience. Create a more positive scenario of a change you can handle.
- **Rewind and stop the fearful movie that replays in your mind.** Imagine you're at a movie theater, and your inner scary movie is going superfast in reverse, with backward voices and the whoosh of the projector. When it's all reversed, imagine the global sign for No (a red circle and slash) across the screen.
- **Remind yourself that you have options.** "I'm imagining one possible future, not the only one."

- **Imagine a new movie of the future you want.**
  Feel yourself in it with sensations in your body.
- **Be grateful for what you have.**

Has Jasmine changed since practicing Positive Focus? She still has the ability to see problems. However, she's more aware now when she's focused on what's wrong and is much better at expressing her gratitude. She sometimes actually lets the problems slide. The salty soup no longer means she should have picked a better restaurant for her fancy night . . . it means she discovered a great new restaurant where she won't order the salty soup. And for that she's also grateful.

Chapter 16

Taking Restful Insomnia Insights into Sleep and the Day

Dreams say what they mean,
but they don't say it in daytime language.
—Gail Godwin

DAYS (EXERCISE, COFFEE, MEDICINE, STRESS) influence your nights. And you know that nights influence your days; that's why you worry at 2:41 A.M. that you'll be zoned out at 2:41 P.M.

Fortunately, Restful Insomnia nights also influence your days. Their influence starts with you resting at 2:41 and extends to your relationship with your body, emotions, Conscious Mind, creativity, and more. And even your relationship to sleep.

My client Natasha was a great sleeper—until she gave birth to her daughter eleven months ago. She'd wake up two or three times a night, change her daughter's diaper, feed her, put her back in her crib . . . and stare at the walls. She'd finally fall asleep a few hours later, just before Victoria cried. Though her husband did much of the child-care duties, he had to be at work early most days. Natasha worried when he helped, instead of resting. She worried that her husband would become overtired, wondered whether she should return to work part-time, start up a freelance graphic business, or stay home with Victoria for the rest of the year. What should her plans be for tomorrow? Should she try to find clients? Her thoughts just kept going.

Restful Insomnia helped unwind the nighttime frenzy. Natasha stayed horizontal as she lay in bed. The sound machine kept her from focusing on her daughter's moves and moans, although she could certainly hear her cry. Between feedings and when her husband was caring for Victoria, she used her eye mask and rolled her eyes down, creating a little cocoon of rest. She had begun to tap into her body and the natural force of life to get some distance from her thoughts.

Once she had those basics down, I talked to her about how to increase the possibility of sleep with Restful Insomnia—not to diminish the benefit of rest, but to add a few actions that would remind her body about snoozing. We also talked about how to use Restful Insomnia during the day—from taking naps to changing her perspective on making decisions about work, marriage, and motherhood.

Return to Sleep? It's Possible

Natasha's connection with her body continued to emerge as she did Restful Insomnia. She could sense—not just in her thoughts, but also in her degree of body tension—whether it was her Conscious Mind or her Unconscious Mind that was driving her mental bus.

Deepening her body awareness could help her monitor when her body was ready to go to sleep. The first sign was immobility. When her Conscious Mind was rattling on about things that needed to be done, she thought she was wide awake. However, if she considered acting on the urges of her mind—say, getting up and checking her e-mail—her body did not want to move. This was one sure indication for her to listen to her body instead of her mind.

As she deepened this awareness, she let go further into sleep. Her mind would wander off onto odd tangents (she was riding a tricycle on a freeway). If she noticed how odd her thoughts were, her Conscious Mind grew uncomfortable. Instead, she focused on her body, breath, or skin.

As sleep neared, Natasha would lose awareness of her body: the little backache from carrying the car seat, the wrinkled pillowcase, a slight sense of being hungry. Of course, once she noticed that she was losing awareness, her mind would rattle awake. Instead of looking at the clock and berating herself for being awake, she would start the cycle again: back into her body, Unconscious Mind, and rest. This time, her mind and body moved into a sleepier state.

Mental Actions

Sometimes Natasha's Conscious Mind was focused on remembering all the tasks to do the next day. Then, Natasha followed my suggestion about using mnemonics. Mnemonics are memory tools that help you remember your shopping list, key points in a chapter, or what to bring to work. By using mnemonics, Natasha wouldn't need to move her body, turn on a light, and write those things down.

To use mnemonics, link what you want to remember to a code. (For instance, you may have learned the colors of the rainbow are "Roy G. Biv"—red, orange, yellow, green, blue, indigo, violet), or link to a phrase, letters, numbers, pictures, songs, or an imagined journey. The more vivid the images and sensations you use, the stronger the association and thus your recollection. For instance, Natasha linked the task of taking clothes to the dry cleaners to the image of a five-foot-tall lime green shirt draped over the door, keeping it from closing. And indeed, when she was closing the door as she got ready to leave the next day, she remembered to get the shirts.

To help mnemonics work better:

- Make the images positive and pleasant, even funny, peculiar, and odd. Exaggerate sizes, colors, and locations.
- Use all your senses—an alarm, dancing objects, a smiling face. Have them crash or merge into each other.

- Associate the object with a usual task you'll do the next day—picturing the three items to return to the store in the bathroom sink.
- Associate the items with easily remembered objects such as traffic lights, road signs, or your body parts. If you need to remember five things, imagine one stuck to your nose, one (with an unusual color) in each of your hands, and one on each of your feet.

Let your Unconscious Mind make the associations while your body rests.

Physical Actions

- **Repeat the Evening Ritual.** If Natasha had to go to the bathroom or get up for Victoria, she'd redo the last steps of her Evening Ritual while keeping her environment fairly dark. She might brush her teeth, put lotion on her feet, or read a book review in *O* magazine. That reminded her Unconscious Mind of the nightly habit that preceded her first few hours of sleep.
- **Use the Night Nest.** Natasha would make sure her sound machine was on, spray some lavender-scented mist, and use the seashell to remind herself of how soothing her vacation was.
- **Experience sexual pleasure.** Sexual release of course focused Natasha on her body and allowed her

tension to dissipate. Not to mention that it got her breathing more deeply.

- **Use an eye mask.** If Natasha hadn't used her eye mask, she'd put it on. Something about that blackness around her eyes reminded her of letting go. Or she'd roll her eyes down again. (They'd unroll when her thoughts were gearing up.) When her eyes naturally rolled up, she knew she was really resting—only she rarely noticed it.

Sleep is wonderful, but worrying about sleep is a race with no reward. Enjoy your rest, and enjoy sleep when it comes.

Using Restful Insomnia During the Day

Natasha found that she could use the new balance of her Conscious Mind and her Unconscious Mind during her days. She used the Restful Insomnia techniques to help her Conscious Mind not run in circles as she tried to be a perfect mom. Instead, she had access to more wisdom to help her out.

- **Restful Insomnia techniques during the day.** Natasha starting making use of moments of meditation to calm herself during the day. She also used the Tapas Acupressure Technique from Energy Psychology when she became stressed by her husband's late hours. Most important, she used Restful Insomnia techniques to take short naps—using an eye mask, a sound machine, and body awareness—when Victoria slept during the day after being up most of the night with a cold.

- **Restful Insomnia insights.** Natasha benefited during the day from doing Wisdom Writing about her work at night. She learned that she didn't have to make a decision immediately, that the timing wasn't right yet. She moved into a relaxed research mode, asking other moms about their experience and networking with former clients to understand current opportunities. She made sure to enjoy the time she had right now with Victoria as her daughter was learning to walk and babbling—just as her deeper wisdom had suggested she do.

- **Spiritual Center.** Natasha hadn't thought much about the spiritual state of the world, but she experienced it after the birth of Victoria. Life had too many miracles to not appreciate the mysteries that made them happen. She valued the permission in Restful Insomnia to create her own relationship with her Spiritual Center, which she called the Natural Force. She wasn't sure whether she believed that all the connections she made were real. She thought some of them were the result of making up a story about deeper harmony in life than she could always see. But it was a pleasant way to live, and she was more connected to giving to others because of it. She felt more balanced and creative, and in touch with the cycle of life, so she'd just consider her Spiritual Center story real. Why not?

The cycle of life endures, with days influencing nights and nights influencing days. Your body wants to surrender when you're lying in bed just wishing for sleep. The key is to find *your* way—just for tonight—to give the Conscious Mind a break, and let the Unconscious Mind steer the night raft. In rest or sleep.

Your way may be the same as last week, or your relationship with the dictating Conscious Mind may require something new: a temporary truce (let's try this just for ten minutes), a distraction (how many traffic lights are there between your house and work?), soothing (you've worked hard, lets talk in the morning), reverse psychology (you couldn't possibly focus on the breath for five minutes), or new focus (what does the roof of the mouth feel like?). If you don't know what you need intuitively, re-read some Restful Insomnia chapters to find methods that suit tonight's body, mind, and environment.

Eventually, the Conscious Mind learns that it *does* need a break—sleep or focus on the Unconscious Mind with Restful Insomnia. When it rests, your body, spirit, emotions, *and* the Conscious Mind enjoy the days as well.

Let me know about your nights and days after you've used Restful Insomnia. You can send me e-mail via my Web site, *www.restfulinsomnia.com,* which includes new tips and a link to my blog. I'll look forward to hearing (in the morning—I need to rest at night!) about what you've gained, even during insomnia.

Enjoy your nights!

Bibliography and Resources

Books

Marianne Binetti. *Easy Answers for Great Gardens: 500 Tips, Techniques and Outlandish Ideas*. Seattle, WA: Sasquatch Books, 2002.

Joan Borysenko. *Minding the Body, Mending the Mind*. Cambridge, MA: Da Capo Press, 2007.

Rick Carson. *Taming Your Gremlin: A Surprisingly Simple Method for Getting Out of Your Own Way*. New York: Quill, 2003.

Gavin de Becker. *The Gift of Fear: And Other Survival Signals That Protect Us from Violence*. New York: Dell, 1999.

Donna Eden. *Energy Medicine: Balance Your Body's Energies for Optimum Health, Joy, and Vitality*. New York: Tarcher/Penguin, 1999.

Tapas Fleming. *You Can Heal Now: The Tapas Acupressure Technique (TAT)*. Redondo Beach, CA: TAT International, 1999.

Shakti Gawain. *Creative Visualization*. Novato, CA: Nataraj Publications/New World Library, 2002.

Bill Hayes. *Sleep Demons: An Insomniac's Memoir*. New York: Washington Square Press, 2001.

Byron Katie. *Loving What Is: Four Questions That Can Change Your Life.* New York: Crown, 2002.

Garrison Keillor. *Good Poems.* New York: Penguin, 2003.

Sally Kempton (Swami Durgananda). *The Heart of Meditation: Pathways to a Deeper Experience.* South Fallsburg, NY: SYDA Foundation, 2002.

Jack Kornfield. *After the Ecstasy, the Laundry: How the Heart Grows Wise on the Spiritual Path.* New York: Bantam Books, 2001.

Jack Kornfield. *Buddha's Little Instruction Book.* New York: Bantam Books, 1994.

Jack Kornfield. *Meditation for Beginners.* Louisville, CO: Sounds True, 2008.

Anne Lamott. *Plan B: Further Thoughts on Faith.* New York: Penguin, 2006.

Judith Lasater. *Relax and Renew: Restful Yoga for Stressful Times.* Berkeley, CA: Rodmell Press, 1995.

Stephen Levine. *A Gradual Awakening.* New York: Knopf Doubleday, 1989.

Stephen Levine. *Unattended Sorrow: Recovering from Loss and Reviving the Heart.* Emmaus, PA: Rodale Press, 2006.

Denise Linn. *Sacred Space.* New York: Random House, 1995.

Ragini Elizabeth Michaels. *Facticity: A Door to Mental Health and Beyond.* Seattle, WA: Facticity Trainings, 1991.

Richard Miller. *Yoga Nidra: The Meditative Heart of Yoga.* Louisville, CO: Sounds True, 2005.

Ronald and Patricia Potter-Efron. *Letting Go of Anger: The Eleven Most Common Anger Styles and What to Do About Them.* Oakland, CA: New Harbinger Publications, 2006.

Lorin Roche. *Meditation Made Easy.* New York: Harper San Francisco, 1998.

Sharon Salzberg. *Faith: Trusting Your Own Deepest Experience.* New York: Penguin, 2003.

Bailey White. *Mama Makes Up Her Mind: And Other Dangers of Southern Living.* Cambridge, MA: Da Capo Press, 2009.

E. B. White. *Charlotte's Web.* New York: HarperCollins, 2006.

Recordings

Osho Deuter. *Active Meditation.* Santa Fe, NM: New Earth Records, 2000.

Ragini Elizabeth Michaels. *The Facticity CD Series: (Beginnings and Endings, Living in Mystery, Balance in Motion, and Trusting).* Seattle, WA: Facticity Trainings (*www.facticity.com*), 2005.

Ragini Elizabeth Michaels. *The Remembrance CD Series: (Beyond the Past, The Healing Heart, Answers Rest Within, and Awareness Rising).* Seattle, WA: Facticity Trainings (*www.facticity.com*), 2005.

Karma Moffett. *Golden Bowls* and *Ocean Bowls.* San Francisco: Padma Music, 2007.

Pure White Noise. *Relaxing River.* Tallahassee, FL: *www. Purewhitenoise.com.*

Shiva Rea. *Drops of Nectar* (includes Yoga Nidra). Boulder, CO: Sounds True, 2002.

Sleep Machines. *Fireplace DVD*. Portland, OR: *www.Sleep machines.com*.

Sleep Machines. *Furnace*. Portland, OR: *www.Sleep machines.com*.

Websites

Babeland.com (women-friendly sex toy shop)

Easternhealth.org.au/champs/images/faces.gif.com (images of different emotions)

Kathewallace.com (physical therapy for pelvic issues)

Purewhitenoise.com (white-noise CDs and MP3 downloads)

Sleepmachines.com (products for sleep and rest)

Tatlife.com (Tapas Acupressure Technique)

Thoughtfieldtherapy.co.uk and *emofree.com* (psychological acupressure)

Virtuesproject.com (strategies that inspire the practice of virtues)

Well.com (for conversation and discussion destination)

And: *RestfulInsomnia.com* for products and blog on the program.

About the Author

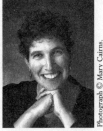

Photograph © Mary Cairns.

Sondra Kornblatt is a health and science writer who developed the Restful Insomnia program in 2000, during a year-long bout of chronic insomnia. Using her experience in visualization, hypnosis, and body awareness, she found methods to relax and renew when sleep was elusive. Sondra is also the author of *A Better Brain at Any Age* and *365 Energy Boosters*. She lives with her family in the Pacific Northwest.

To Our Readers

Conari Press, an imprint of Red Wheel/Weiser, publishes books on topics ranging from spirituality, personal growth, and relationships to women's issues, parenting, and social issues. Our mission is to publish quality books that will make a difference in people's lives—how we feel about ourselves and how we relate to one another. We value integrity, compassion, and receptivity, both in the books we publish and in the way we do business.

Our readers are our most important resource, and we value your input, suggestions, and ideas about what you would like to see published. Please feel free to contact us, to request our latest book catalog, or to be added to our mailing list.

Conari Press
An imprint of Red Wheel/Weiser, LLC
500 Third Street, Suite 230
San Francisco, CA 94107
www.redwheelweiser.com